STELLA PAK, MD

UNIQUE INSIGHT

Seeing Scripture from an Autistic Point of View

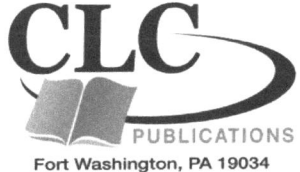

Fort Washington, PA 19034

Unique Insight
Published by CLC Publications

USA: P.O. Box 1449, Fort Washington, PA 19034
www.clcpublications.com

UK: Kingsway CLC Trust
Unit 5, Glendale Avenue, Sandycroft, Flintshire, CH5 2QP
www.equippingthechurch.com

© 2024 Stella Pak
All rights reserved. Published 2024

For permission to reprint, please contact us at:
permissions@clcpublications.com

Printed in the United States of America

ISBN (paperback): 978-1-61958-398-6
ISBN (e-book): 978-1-61958-399-3

Unless otherwise noted, Scripture quotations are from the Lexham English Bible, Copyright © 2012 by Logos Bible Software. Lexham is a registered trademark of Logos Bible Software. All rights reserved worldwide.

Italics in Scripture quotations, if not original to the LEB, are the emphasis of the author.

PRAISE FOR
UNIQUE INSIGHT

In *Unique Insight*, Dr. Pak, a physician and devoted Christian, crafts a captivating debut devotional. She transports us to the era of the Bible's writing, inviting us to imagine the context and glean practical takeaways for our lives. Dr. Pak's medical background in autism guides the book's application of the ABC and FAST methods. They prove valuable for autistic readers as well as everyone else. This book was refreshing and insightful to read. I have never read a book quite like it.

— Robert J. Nash
Pastor at Sawyer Highlands and
Converge Community Church, Sawyer, MI

As a professor of theology and license minister diagnosed with autism, I process information literally and I am a visual thinker. While studying the Bible in college this created challenges with interpreting abstract concepts, motifs, social contexts, and metaphors. Autism made me feel like a social leper, but with love, acceptance, and faith in Christ, I experienced a sense of belonging. *Unique Insight: Seeing Scripture from an Autistic Point of View* is the perfect guide to empower our faith by providing a hermeneutical approach to a deeper understanding of biblical passages, making them relatable and resonant with the autistic reader. I highly recommend Dr. Stella Pak's book to every person with autism who desires to enrich their relationship with Christ by interpreting and applying the Scriptures and church leaders and educators with a passion for inclusion.

— Ron Sandison, MDiv
Founder of Spectrum Inclusion and author of
*Views from the Spectrum: A Window into Life
and Faith with Your Neurodivergent Child*

The Bible can be considered a road map to our lives, a way to navigate through the ups and downs that we may experience along our journey of life. It provides parables, interesting characters, moral guideposts, but most of all the saving knowledge of our Lord and Savior Jesus Christ and how we can receive eternal salvation. This is a message that is meant for all to see, hear, and understand. This fantastic new book, *Unique Insight* by Stella Pak, is helping open new doors and making this a possibility within the autistic community. Autism is a challenging disorder that is becoming more and more prominent within the world's population. They struggle to fit in with society, and at times understand basic concepts. Miss Pak has taken stories from the Bible and broken each one of them down so an individual with autism can not only understand the basic concepts of the story, but also be able to see and experience God's love unfolding through these pages and stories so they too can experience the most precious gift we can ever receive—the knowledge and love of our Lord and Savior Jesus Christ! This is a must read and a wonderful experience for all!

— Rev. Dr. David John Scott Quel
Instructor of Special Needs Ministry at the Southwestern College

Written by and for autistic adults, Stella Pak breaks down the stories and metaphors of Scripture into clear and concrete definitions paired with practical action steps. *Unique Insight* makes the Bible accessible to autistic readers in a way that marvelously encourages concrete and real-world ventures of faith.

— Dr. Brian Brock
Professor of Moral and Practical Theology
School of Divinity, History and Philosophy
University of Aberdeen, United Kingdom

Contents

Preface 7

Introduction 9

1. The Braveheart—Ezra 15
2. Naboth's Verdant Vineyard 23
3. The Daughter under His "Wings" 31
4. A Legacy of Faithfulness—Manasseh 37
5. A Legacy of Impiety—Ahab 43
6. The Highways to Zion 47
7. From the Tax Ladder to the Heavenly Elevator—Zacchaeus ... 53
8. Life, Death, and Re-Nain-ssance 61
9. Bed and Bible (B&B) —Gaius 67
10. One Touch of Heaven on the Untouchable 73
11. The Judgement of Solomon 77
12. The First Judge of Israel—Othniel 85
13. The Unlikeliest Rescuer—Jonah's Mission to the Enemy 93
14. Faith in Practice, Part 1:
    Triumphing over Trials—James the Just 107
15. Faith in Practice, Part 2:
    Connecting Belief to Action—James the Just 117

16. Beware the Wolves 125

17. Blessed Beyond Measure—Abraham 129

18. The Invincible Hero of God—Asa 137

19. The Shield of Faith—David 147

20. The Repurposed—Jeremiah 151

21. Faith in the Fire—Peter 157

22. A Little Leaven Leavens the Whole Batch of Dough—Jude .. 163

23. Guided by the Fear of God 171

24. Singing Under the Stars—The Levites 177

25. The Kingdom United—Unity, Love, Peace 181

26. Vanity of Vanity—The Preacher and Paul 185

27. The Sovereign Ruler—Yahweh 191

28. A Man Spared by Divine Providence—Baruch..................... 195

29. Locust Locos: A Loud Call for Repentance—Joel 209

30. Rising Stars of Faith:
    Stories of Exemplary New Christians—The Thessalonians 215

31. The Feast of Remnants—Haggai.. 221

32. Christ Quest, Part 1:
    Spreading the Gospel Against All Odds—Paul...................... 231

33. Christ Quest, Part 2:
    Faith, Hope, and the Second Coming—Paul 243

34. The First Gospel Messenger—-Anna..................................... 251

35. Behold: Unveiling the Son of God—Jesus of Nazareth 257

Appendix: ABC Exercise Dictionary 263

Preface

HAVING AUTISM spectrum disorder, I've often found the Bible to be incredibly challenging to understand. It is filled with abstract, indirect, and subtle expressions as well as numerous allegories, metaphors, parables, parallels, innuendos, sarcasm, and satirical elements, all of which are difficult for people who are on the spectrum to comprehend. The intricate psychological, social, and emotional situations in the stories add another layer of complexity.

As I struggled to comprehend the Scriptures, I had a moment of despair. I began to doubt my place as one of the chosen, questioning whether I was the intended audience for these Scriptures. Then I stumbled upon James 1:5, which says, "Now if any of you lacks wisdom, let him ask for *it* from God, who gives to all without reservation and not reproaching, and it will be given to him." I prayed for divine wisdom to guide me in understanding His word so that I could know who He is. He granted me the strength and patience to dive deep into the Scriptures. Through practice, I developed a skill set that allowed me to translate abstract scriptural concepts into concrete, relatable terms.

Just as the Bible needs to be translated into a person's native language for it to be understandable, so the Bible needs to be adapted into an accessible version for autistic individuals. The skills presented in this book help autistic individuals like me "translate" the Bible into a version that is more understandable for us. A significant advantage of these skills is their applicability for autistic individuals across various linguistic and cultural boundaries.

I have been ecstatic about how these techniques have enriched my own understanding of the Scriptures as well as how they have helped other autistic individuals. Surprisingly, even those without autism have found these methods beneficial in achieving a deeper understanding of biblical passages. While learning these skills, they have developed an understanding of how autism influences the processing of information. This invaluable insight has helped them to connect and communicate more effectively with autistic Christians. This foundational understanding has also enabled them to assist and support autistic Christians in their Bible studies. These changes have cultivated a more inclusive and supportive environment for autistic Christians within their church communities.

Encouraged by their positive impacts, I've expanded these skills into a book to introduce them to a broader Christian audience, including autistic and non-autistic readers. My hope is that these techniques will not only deepen people's understanding of the Bible but also promote unity among autistic and non-autistic Christians. I also hope this book can pave the path toward greater acceptance and integration of autistic Christians within church communities.

Best Regards,
Stella Pak, MD

Introduction
"Unique" Bible Reading Skills and Their Application for Autistic Readers

AUTISM SPECTRUM disorders (ASD) encompass a range of conditions where individuals experience distinct ways of processing information across various cognitive domains. These conditions may affect how individuals perceive, understand, and interact with the world around them.[1] Challenges in communication and social interactions associated with autism often arise not only from the characteristics of the disorder itself but also from societal factors such as a lack of awareness, tolerance, support, and advocacy for autistic individuals.[2]

Within closely knit church communities, autistic Christians often feel excluded due to difficulties in navigating social interactions. The struggle to integrate into the church community, along with preaching and teaching that is often inaccessible to them, makes it hard for autistic individuals to understand God's teachings and live a faith-centered life. These difficulties highlight the necessity of Scripture-reading strategies tailored for autistic

---

1 M.K. Belmonte, E.H. Cook Jr., G.M. Anderson, et al., "Autism as a disorder of neural information processing: directions for research and targets for therapy," *Molecular Psychiatry* 9 (7): 646–663 (2004).

2 R.R. Grinker, "Autism, 'Stigma,' Disability: A Shifting Historical Terrain," *Current Anthropology* 61 (S21): S55–S67 (2020).

Christians. Increasing accessibility to God's Word would empower autistic Christians to stand firm in their faith despite the adversities they face in their spiritual life.

People with ASD often struggle to understand abstract ideas and concepts.[3] The Bible, with its numerous abstract concepts like righteousness and faith, can be an overwhelming challenge. To tackle this specific issue, we include two tools at the end of every chapter in this book: the **ABC** (**A**bstract to **B**rick **C**oncrete) and **FAST** (**F**ocused, **A**ctionable **S**teps to **T**ake). These skill sets aid autistic readers—and others, as well—in systematically translating abstract concepts into more practical and tangible terms.

The ABC skill involves translating an abstract concept into concrete and tangible terms using relevant biblical passages, then comparing it to the general dictionary definition. This approach makes the concept less ambiguous and more comprehensible.

The next exercise, called the FAST skill, involves constructing practical and actionable steps drawn from insights found in biblical passages. Each step is supported by specific and tangible examples applied to everyday life. The ABC and FAST skill sets bridge the gap between abstract concepts and practical implementation, helping autistic individuals to study the Bible more effectively.

Autism can also make it challenging to grasp the details of various social contexts.[4] To assist the reader in overcoming this, we provide thorough information on the social context, historical background, and cultural nuances of each biblical passage.

---

3   D. Ropar, D. Peebles, "Sorting preference in children with autism: The dominance of concrete features," *Journal of Autism and Developmental Disorders* 37 (2): 270–280 (2007).

4   R.P. Lawson, J. Aylward, J.P. Roiser, G. Rees, "Adaptation of social and non-social cues to direction in adults with autism spectrum disorder and neurotypical adults with autistic traits," *Developmental Cognitive Neuroscience* 29: 108–116 (2018).

Some autistic individuals might not readily relate to the mental and emotional experiences of characters in stories or narratives.[5] To enhance the relatability of the biblical passages, we provide detailed descriptions of the psychological perspectives within each narrative.

Autism manifests itself differently in each person, with varying symptoms and levels of intensity.[6] The strategies introduced in this book are designed to address symptoms most frequently associated with autism: concrete thinking, reduced empathy, and diminished social awareness.

While such an approach may work for many autistic Christians, it may not be suitable for everyone. For an autistic Christian whose needs don't fully align with the strategies outlined in this book, I strongly urge you to openly discuss your specific challenges in Scripture reading with both healthcare providers and respected church leaders. Collaboration between healthcare professionals and church leaders is critical in addressing the spiritual needs of individuals with less typical manifestations of ASD.

Unleashing Unique Insight *for All Readers*

Unique Insight invites readers to experience the Bible from an unconventional angle, through the lens of autism. It takes a highly literal approach, thoroughly examining the actual words in the Bible for its straightforward and factual interpretation.[7] This approach minimizes confusion or misinterpretation that may arise from allegorical analysis, where symbolic or metaphorical

---

5 Irene E. Harmsen, "Empathy in Autism Spectrum Disorder," *Journal of Autism and Developmental Disorders* 49 (10): 3939–3955 (2019).

6 A. Masi, M.M. DeMayo, N. Glozier, et al., "An Overview of Autism Spectrum Disorder, Heterogeneity and Treatment Options," *Neuroscience Bulletin* 33: 183–193 (2017).

7 Augustin Vicente, Christian Michel, and Valentine Petrolini, "Literalism in Autistic People: a Predictive Processing Proposal," *Review of Philosophy and Psychology*, 2023.

meanings are arbitrarily applied. Examining the actual text also serves to limit the influence of speculative or subjective views in understanding the Bible.

It also brings a fresh, unconventional perspective to the study of the Bible, offering distinctive interpretations and insights. This perspective likely stems from a reduced tendency to conform to societal and cultural norms, a key trait of autism.[8] This atypical inclination ironically serves to safeguard the interpretation of the Scriptures from social or cultural biases.

Throughout its pages, the Bible depicts social outcasts—lepers, widows, orphans, shepherds, tax collectors, and sojourners—echoing experiences familiar to individuals with autism.[9] Rooted in personal experiences of social exclusion, individuals with autism can deeply relate to the thoughts, emotions, and circumstances mirrored in the social outcasts portrayed in the biblical passages. Through this autistic lens, readers can step into the characters' shoes, feeling the heartbeat of these narratives, making the biblical passages profoundly relatable and resonant.

Autistic individuals often demonstrate exceptional attention to detail and intense focus. These cognitive tendencies drive thorough exploration of biblical passages, resulting in an incredibly in-depth analysis of the Bible.[10] Through this robust

---

8 Sarah Woods and Annette Estes, "Toward a more comprehensive autism assessment: the survey of autistic strengths, skills, and interests," *Frontiers in Psychiatry* 14: 1264516 (2023).

9 Laura Hull, K.V. Petride, Carrie Allison, Paula Smith, Simon Baron-Cohen, Meng-Chuan Lai and Mandy William, "'Putting on My Best Normal': Social Camouflaging in Adults with Autism Spectrum Conditions," *Journal of Autism and Developmental Disorders* 47 (8): 2519–2534 (2017).

10 Francesca Happé and Pedro Vital, "What aspects of autism predispose to talent?" *Philosophical Transactions of the Royal Society of London*, Series B, Biological Sciences, 364 (1522): 1369–75 (2009).

analysis, critical but often overlooked details come to the forefront, illuminating aspects that enrich the overall comprehension of the Bible.

Let's look now at some examples of how to apply these techniques to studying the Scripture so that you can learn by doing.

1

The Braveheart—Ezra

This Ezra went up from Babylonia. He was a scribe skilled in the law of Moses, which Yahweh the God of Israel gave. The king granted him all his requests, for the hand of Yahweh was upon him. . . . For Ezra had set his heart to seek the law of Yahweh, to do it, *and to teach the regulations and judgments in Israel.*

Ezra 7:6, 10

AARON PASSED DOWN the high priesthood through generations (Ezra 7:1–5; 1 Chron. 6:3–15), with Phinehas and Zadok notably known for their exceptional holy zeal and righteousness. The high priesthood was later bestowed upon Jehozadak (Hag. 1:1), who had a brother named Ezra (1 Chron. 6:14; Ezra 7:1). The name *Ezra* means "help," which perfectly described him as a man who walked with the helping hand of God upon him. He displayed an unwavering dedication to wholeheartedly study, obey, and teach God's words, in sync with his mission statement found in 7:10: "For Ezra had set his heart to seek the law of Yahweh, to do *it*, and to teach the regulations and judgments in Israel." Endowed with divine wisdom, he rose to the position of a scribe overseeing Jewish affairs, a role analogous to that of a chancellor or secretary of state.[1] Additionally, through God's divine intervention, the King of Persia became a staunch supporter of Ezra, granting his every request with enthusiasm.

> Artaxerxes, the king of kings, to Ezra the priest, the scribe of the law of the God of the heavens. Peace. And now I issue forth a decree that any of the people of Israel, their priests, or their Levites in my kingdom who are willing to go to Jerusalem may go with you. For you are sent from the king and his seven counselors to enquire about Judah and Jerusalem concerning the law of your God, which is in your hand. . . .
>
> You, Ezra, according to the wisdom of your God that you possess, appoint magistrates and judges who can judge all of the people *in the province* Beyond the River who know the laws of your God. And you will teach those who do not know. All who do not obey the law of your God and the law of the king, let judgment be executed on him with diligence, whether for death or for banishment or for confiscation of goods and for imprisonment. (Ezra 7:12–14, 25–26)
>
> You *must observe them* [the laws of God] *diligently*, for that is your wisdom and your insight before the eyes of the people, who will hear all *of* these rules, and they will say, "Surely this great nation *is* a wise and discerning people." (Deut. 4:6)

His unwavering faith not only inspired the Israelites but also touched the hearts of pagan Gentiles in the Persian Empire. This admiration is evident in the letter from the Persian King Artaxerxes, where he referred to Ezra as the "scribe [chancellor] of the law of the God of the heavens" (7:12). God chose this man whose heart was bound to His sacred Word to spearhead the second return of the remnant of the Israelites from Babylon to Jerusalem. According to the divine providence, King Artaxerxes

---

[1] Karel Van-Der-Toorn, *Scribal Culture and the Making of the Hebrew Bible* (Cambridge, MA: Harvard University Press, 2009), 77–79.

granted Ezra full authority to institute a governmental system in the kingdom of Judah. Alongside this decree, the king gave permission to the Jews who desired to go to Jerusalem to follow Ezra on his journey.

In Deuteronomy 4:6, Moses proclaimed that wisdom arises from diligently studying and obeying God's words. This truth was affirmed in the life of Ezra as the wisdom of God manifested in him through divine inspiration. In Ezra 7:25, the pagan King Artaxerxes I, who reigned over the Persian Empire, astonishingly disclosed his observation that Ezra's wisdom flowed from his wholehearted dedication to the laws of his God, Yahweh. This revelation illuminates the awe-inspiring depth of Ezra's wisdom and casts a spotlight on the transcendent impact of his holy zeal. The influence of Ezra was so extraordinary that it compelled a pagan king to humbly recognize the God of Israel. He not only acknowledged the legitimacy of Ezra's divine quest but, in a resounding declaration, bore witness to Yahweh as the true God.

> Also, bring the silver and gold that the king and his advisors have freely offered to the God of Israel whose dwelling is in Jerusalem, and all of the silver and gold that you will find in the whole province of Babylonia, with the freewill offerings of the people and the priests giving willingly for the house of their God in Jerusalem. . . .
>
> I weighed out into their hand six hundred and fifty talents of silver, one hundred vessels of silver, one hundred talents of gold, twenty gold bowls worth one thousand darics, and two vessels of good polished bronze as precious as gold. (Ezra 7:15–16; 8:26–27)
>
> I have sworn by myself; a word that shall not return has gone forth from my mouth *in* righteousness: "Every knee shall kneel down to me; every tongue shall swear." (Isa. 45:23)
>
> For he will be like a tree planted by water, and to *the* stream it sends its roots, and it will not fear when heat comes, and its

leaves will be luxuriant, and in *the* year of drought it will not be anxious, and it will not cease from the bearing of fruit. (Jer. 17:8)

Ezra was also entrusted with an immense wealth of silver, gold, and vessels for the Temple service in Jerusalem, collectively valued at over three million dollars.[2] These precious offerings, bestowed by the king, his advisors, and the common people in their devotion, clearly demonstrate the profound divine recognition of Yahweh in the Empire of Persia.

This fulfillment of the Scriptures, echoing the prophecy of Isaiah 45:23, where foreign nations bow down to Yahweh, serves as a powerful testament to His boundless magnificence. Even amid the Babylonian captivity, He received the utmost honor from all nations, affirming His eternal sovereignty. This established His supremacy over the pagan idol gods, whose influence was limited by the status and deeds of their followers.

Devout followers of Yahweh, like Ezra, were elevated, honored, and blessed in a land steeped in wickedness, injustice, and pagan idol worship. Just as an evergreen tree draws life-sustaining water from the river, Ezra nurtured himself with the life-giving words of God. Even amid drought, those rooted by the riverbank remain in verdant glory, untouched by the scorching heat. Similarly, Ezra clung to God's words, thriving without being affected by the trials of exile. His unwavering faith and wholehearted commitment to God's word earned him respect, reverence, and ultimately, a divine wisdom.

> I proclaimed a fast there at the river Ahava to humble ourselves before our God in order to seek from him a safe journey for us, our children, and our possessions. For I was ashamed to ask the king for troops and horses to protect us from enemies on the way because we said to the king, "the hand of our God is favorable to all who seek him, but his strength

---

[2] Charles Foster Kent, *The Makers and Teachers of Judaism* (McFarland, WI: Books on Demand, 2020), 121.

and anger are against all who forsake them." So we fasted and sought our God for this and he responded to our prayer. . . .

On the twelfth day of the first month we set out from the river of Ahava to go to Jerusalem. The hand of our God was on us and he delivered us from the hand of the enemy and from ambushing on the way. (Ezra 8:21–23, 31)

Ezra set out to guide the remnant on a grueling four-month, 900-mile journey back to Jerusalem. It was a treacherous road, infested with ruthless bandits and lurking thieves. The caravan of remnants consisted of approximately 5,000 Israelites, with men making up only 20 percent of the total—the majority were women, children, and the elderly.[3] This demographic composition, combined with their invaluable cargo, made them an exceedingly attractive target for bandits, plunderers, and brigands. In the face of peril, Ezra made a resolute choice, a choice that defined his unyielding faith. With a holy zeal for God, he spurned the idea of seeking an armed escort. To him, such a request would not only be an affront to his unwavering trust in the Almighty but a dishonor to the very name of God. He felt shame at the mere thought of relying on mortal hands when he had consistently declared his trust in the good hand of God upon him. Instead, with heads bowed and spirits humbled, Ezra and the remnants turned to God. In the sacred silence of fasting and the fervency of prayer, they beseeched God for divine guidance and protection. Their heart pulsated with holy zeal to proclaim Yahweh as the sole redeemer for the Israelites.

The good hand of God was undoubtedly upon Ezra and the remnants during their journey. They enjoyed good health and security throughout this lengthy and challenging expedition. God's providence guided, directed, and protected them every

---

[3] Stan Purdum, *Immersion Bible Studies: Ezra, Nehemiah, Esther* (Nashville: Abingdon Press, 2013), 21–30.

step of the way. The safe passage of thousands of people on this arduous odyssey stands out as one of the most remarkable events in history. This extraordinary journey, a testament to divine intervention, resonated not only with the survivors but also brought great glory to God, captivating the attention of nations far and wide.

The decision by Ezra to not ask a pagan king for an armed escort was similar to a decision by Abram (later named Abraham) to not accept a share in the spoils of war from a pagan king.

> Abram said to the king of Sodom, "I have raised my hand to Yahweh, God Most High, Maker of heaven and earth, *that neither a thread nor* a thong of a sandal would I take from all that *belongs* to you, that you might not say, 'I made Abram rich.'" (Gen. 14:22–23)

After Abraham achieved a momentous victory in the battle of Siddim, rescuing Sodom, Gomorrah, and their allies, King Bera of Sodom graciously offered Abraham the spoils he had acquired in the war. However, Abraham, with unyielding faith in God's promise to make him enormously wealthy, declined the offer. He did not want to dishonor God by accepting human help as if God's assistance were insufficient to fulfill his destiny.

Both Abraham and Ezra demonstrated a deep concern for how their actions might either honor or dishonor the name of Yahweh. They prioritized His honor over their own reputation, safety, or worldly success. Their holy zeal for His glory and honor propelled them to live up to the bold faith they professed throughout their lives.

The ABC (Abstract to Brick Concrete)
Holy Zeal—General Definition:[4]

- *Holy*: Exalted or worthy of complete devotion as one perfect in goodnesss and righteousness; devoted entirely to the deity or the work of the deity; having a divine quality; venerated as or as if sacred.
- *Zeal*: Eagerness and ardent interest in pursuit of something.

Holy Zeal—Biblical Definition:

- Unyielding determination to ensure that one's own actions do not obscure God's glory, but instead make it manifest to the entire world.

The FAST (Focused, Actionable Steps to Take)

Integrate and exercise your faith in your everyday actions to glorify God. This means aligning your words and actions with the teachings of Christ. By practicing this, you become a living testament to your faith.

Example: Every Saturday, Tom volunteers at a local homeless shelter, not just serving meals, but also sitting down with those in need. He listens to their stories, offers words of encouragement, and prays with them if they wish. His dedication to this service exemplifies holy zeal. God's love and compassion shine through this exercise of faith.

---

4 "Holy," "Zeal," Merriam-Webster.com, accessed October 23, 2023, https://www.merriam-webster.com.

2

Naboth's Verdant Vineyard

Joseph is the bough of a fruitful vine, a fruitful bough by a spring. His branches climb over the wall.

Genesis 49:22

Manasseh and Ephraim, whom Asenath, daughter of Potiphera, priest of On bore to him, were born to Joseph in the land of Egypt.

Genesis 46:20

ON HIS DEATHBED, Jacob bestowed his blessing upon Joseph and his descendants, praying for their vineyards to flourish with bountiful grapevines, their branches extending over walls. Manasseh, the firstborn son of Joseph, saw his descendants multiply abundantly, ultimately coalescing into the mighty tribe of Manasseh. Jacob's blessing came to fruition as the vineyards tended by the people of Manasseh flourished with lush and verdant grapevines.

> Then the allotment was made for the tribe of Manasseh, because he *was* the firstborn of Joseph. To Makir, the firstborn of Manasseh, the father of Gilead, *were allotted* Gilead and Bashan, because he was a warrior. (Josh. 17:1)

Naboth, whose name means "fruit," was a Menashite who owned a prosperous vineyard located in the outskirts of the city of Jezeel.[1] As the fifth generation tending the lush vineyard, he cherished it as the fulfillment of Jacob's divine blessing. He regarded it not as his personal property, but as a sacred gift and responsibility from God—a divine inheritance.

> The fourth allotment *fell* for Issachar, for the descendants of Issachar, according to their families. Their border went to Jezreel, Chesulloth, Shunem. (19:17–18)

King Ahab of Israel, an Issacharite, owned the city of Jezreel, which bordered the vineyard of Naboth. Ahab gazed from his palace upon the flourishing vineyard adjacent to his home. Instead of recognizing it as a divine blessing, he attributed its abundance solely to the fertile soil. The fertility of the land fueled his greed, leading him to covet the vineyard. He desired to claim the land for his personal garden, cultivating a variety of vegetables and herbs. The herbs were intended for making fragrant incense, but their purpose was to worship the pagan idol gods Baal and Asherah.

> Naboth the Jezreelite had a vineyard which *was* in Jezreel beside the palace of Ahab king of Samaria. Ahab spoke to Naboth, saying, "Give me your vineyard that it may be mine for a garden of vegetable plants, because it is near, beside my house, and I will give to you a better vineyard in place of it. If it is better in your eyes, I will give you the money for its price." Naboth said to Ahab, "Far be it from me from Yahweh [the LORD forbid, ESV] that I should give the inheritance of my ancestors to you." (1 Kings 21:1–3)

---

[1] Thomas Inman, *Ancient Faiths Embodied in Ancient Names*, Vol. I (Frankfurt, Germany: Anatiposi Verlag, 2023), 125.

King Ahab approached Naboth, offering to purchase his vineyard with money or to exchange it for a superior one. Yet, Naboth resolutely invoked God's law, which forbade the transfer of land between individuals from different tribes, reminding the king of this sacred prohibition (Lev. 25:15, 23, 25; Num. 36:7). Furthermore, Naboth could not allow the land of divine blessing to be misused for the worship of pagan idols and gods.

> Ahab went to his house, sullen and angry because of the word that Naboth the Jezreelite had spoken to him *when* he had said, "I will not give to you the inheritance of my ancestors." So he lay on his bed, turned away his face, and would not eat *any* food. Then Jezebel his wife came to him, and she said to him, "What is this, that your spirit is sullen and you are not eating food?" Then he said to her, "When I spoke to Naboth the Jezreelite and asked him, 'Give me your vineyard for money, or if you prefer, I will give you a vineyard in place of it,' he said, 'I will not give you my vineyard.'" Jezebel his wife said to him, "Now, you *rule* over Israel. Get up, eat food, and let your heart be *cheerful*. I myself will give you the vineyard of Naboth the Jezreelite." (1 Kings 21:4–7)

King Ahab does not employ force or coercion to obtain the vineyard, which implies his recognition of the legitimacy of Naboth's ownership and his right to refuse. In his heart, Ahab grapples with conflicting forces—his desire for the vineyard, driven by covetousness, and his recognition that Naboth's refusal was morally and legally right. In an attempt to reconcile his covetous yearning with this inner recognition, he resorts to subtly distorting Naboth's words as below:

Original Statement: "Far be it from me from Yahweh [the LORD forbid, ESV] that I should give the inheritance of my ancestors to you."

First Rendition: "I will not give to you the inheritance of my ancestors."

Second Rendition: "I will not give you my vineyard."

As Ahab progressively reinterprets Naboth's original refusal, it loses its moral and religious validity, appearing increasingly arbitrary. The altered statement falsely paints Naboth as a man of rebellion and disdain for the king. Ahab's kingship faced continuous scrutiny due to the circumstances of his father Omri's rise to power, which involved a civil war in Israel, the death of the previous king, Zimri, and the killing of Omri's rival for the throne, Tibni (1 Kings 16:15–22). In this context, it prompted Jezebel to take decisive action to publicly reinforce Ahab's kingship.

> So she wrote letters in the name of Ahab and sealed them with his seal. She sent the letters to the elders and the nobles who *were* dwelling with Naboth in his city. She had written in the letters, saying, "Call a fast and seat Naboth at the head of the people. Seat two men, *scoundrels*, opposite him. Let them witness against him saying, 'You cursed God and the king.' Then you shall bring him out and stone him so that he dies." The men of his city and the elders and nobles who were living in his city did according to what Jezebel had sent to them, as *was* written in the letters which she had sent to them. They called a fast, and they seated Naboth at the head of the people. Then the two men, *scoundrels*, came, sat opposite him, and the *scoundrels* witnessed against Naboth before the people, saying, "Naboth cursed God and the king," so they brought him outside of the city and stoned him with stones, and he died. (21:8–13)
>
> "Since I saw the blood of Naboth and the blood of his children yesterday," declares Yahweh, "I will requite it for you in this tract of land," declares Yahweh. (2 Kings 9:26)

Jezebel orchestrated a malicious plot that falsely framed Naboth as a traitor, accusing him of blasphemy against both God and the king of Israel. This sinister scheme not only led to Naboth's unjust execution by stoning at the hands of the elders and nobles but also extended its wicked grasp to his sons, ensuring they wouldn't assert their rightful claim of inheritance to the vineyard. Amid her fervent idol worship, she stoned a righteous man faithful to Yahweh, all on charges of blasphemy. This glaring irony unveils the depths of her wickedness and abuse of authority.

> They sent to Jezebel saying, "Naboth has been stoned, and he is dead." It happened at the moment Jezebel heard that Naboth had been stoned and died, Jezebel said to Ahab, "Get up, take possession of the vineyard of Naboth the Jezreelite which he had refused to give to you for money, for Naboth is not alive, but dead." When Ahab heard that Naboth was dead, he got up to go down to the vineyard of Naboth the Jezreelite to take possession of it. (1 Kings 21:14–16)

When Jezebel announced Naboth's death and offered Ahab the vineyard, his response unfurled his chilling manipulation concealed beneath a mask of innocence. Without hesitation, he rushed to take possession of the vineyard as soon as he heard the news. Despite Jezebel's active role, Ahab was the puppeteer behind the scenes, fully immersed in the vile act.

King Ahab displayed a callous disregard for the life of the righteous man of Israel, Naboth. He failed to grasp the profound responsibility that came with his role as the sovereign of Israel. To him, the lives of the Israelites were mere chattels, akin to his view of Naboth's vineyard, which he regarded not as a sacred legacy from God but as a personal possession. In his actions, he betrayed a lack of recognition for the Israelites as the cherished covenant people of Yahweh.

This account serves as a poignant reminder of the importance of recognizing and cherishing the responsibilities and gifts God has bestowed upon us. Likewise, we should honor and respect the divinely given blessings and responsibilities of others.

The ABC (Abstract to Brick Concrete)

Possession—General Definition:[2]

- Ownership; something owned, occupied, or controlled.

Possession—Biblical Definition:

- Divine blessings and responsibilities granted by God for our time on Earth, to be managed with care and gratitude.

The FAST (Focused, Actionable Steps to Take)

1. Foster a deep and lasting sense of gratitude, drawing inspiration from Naboth's profound appreciation for the divine gifts he received from God. His example serves as a reminder not to treat these entrusted resources as mere personal properties but to cherish them as precious gifts intended for our well-being and the support of fellow Christians.

   Example: Anna's daily routine involves writing down her expressions of gratitude to God. She takes the time to note what she is thankful for, with her financial blessings being a significant part of her reflections. Additionally, she offers direct thanks to God through prayers of gratitude that she integrates into her weekly routines.

2. Practice responsible resource management as both a duty and an expression of gratitude to God. Wisely handle the wealth and possessions entrusted to you by budgeting and planning your finances. Ensure that what you've been given is thoughtfully used to support your needs, fulfill your commitments, and assist those in need.

   Example 1: Peter has accumulated a certain amount of wealth, but instead of spending it on his own pleasure, he

---

[2] "Possession," Merriam-Webster.com, accessed October 23, 2023, https://www.merriam-webster.com.

practices responsible stewardship of his financial resources. He does not engage in a lavish lifestyle of opulent homes, costly vehicles, or extravagant pursuits. Instead, he invests a substantial amount of his finances in a Christian senior care facility that offers not only physical support but also spiritual nourishment. He hires chaplains to lead Sunday services, conduct Bible study groups, and offer prayer to the residents and their loved ones. He also sponsors ministries that bring God's Word to rural or remote areas with limited access to religious resources.

Example 2: Fred, a professional financial advisor, is deeply committed to assisting fellow Christians in the wise stewardship of the financial resources granted by God. He conducts workshops on financial literacy, budgeting, and investment. These sessions equip individuals with practical financial knowledge, ensuring their financial decisions align with their faith and responsible principles.

3

The Daughter under His "Wings"

Speak to the Israelites, *and tell them to make for themselves tassels on the hems of their garments [*kanaph*] throughout their generations and to put a blue cord on the tassel of the hem [*kanaph*]. You will have a tassel* **for you to look at** *and remember all the commands of Yahweh and do them, and not follow* **after the unfaithfulness of your own heart and eyes,** *so that you will remember and do all my commandments, and you will be holy for your God.*

Numbers 15:38–40

G OD PROVIDED the Israelites with instructions to wear tassels on the hems of their garments, serving as a physical reminder of His commandments. These tassels, known as *tzitzit*, were a distinct feature of the garments worn by the Israelites, setting them apart as God's chosen people.

In Numbers 15:38, the Hebrew word *kanaph* was used to refer to the hem of garments, but in other places it was translated as "corner," "border," "edge," or "wings." With the passage of time, *kanaph* also came to signify the *tzitzit* (ritual tassels) due to its location on the corners of the garments.[1]

> But for you who revere my name, the sun of righteousness will rise, with healing in its wings [*kanaph*], and you will go out and leap like *fattened calves*. (Mal. 4:2)

The "Sun of Righteousness" in Malachi 4:2 is a scriptural Messianic title that finds fulfillment in Jesus Christ.[2] This title alludes to the Messiah's role in ushering in everlasting righteousness, with all his believers receiving justification through faith in Him (Rom. 3:21–26). This christological reference designates this verse as a prophecy about the Messiah.

In Malachi, *kanaph* (which referred to the hem of garments in Numbers 15:38) was translated as "wings" (Mal. 4:2). This messianic prophecy led many Jews at the time to interpret the "wings" as the tassels attached to the hem of the Messiah's garment, fostering a widespread belief in their healing power.[3] The tassels, also known as *tzitzit*, hold a unique place of privacy and sacredness for Jewish men, serving as a tool for their intimate connection with God.[4]

The Greek word that corresponds to *kanaph* also plays a role in a New Testament passage.

> And a woman who was *suffering from hemorrhages* for twelve years (who, *although she* had spent all *her* assets on physicians, was not able to be healed by anyone) came up behind *him and*

---

1 Ninan Madathilparampil-Mammen, *Secrets of the Prayer Shawl* (Self-published [Lulu.com], 2018), 34–36.

2 Mark Allen Hahlen and Clay Alan Ham, *Minor Prophets Volume 2: Nahum-Malachi* (Joplin, MO: College Press, 2006), 576.

3 Ninan Madathilparampil-Mammen, 34–36.

4 Jay Michaelson, *God in Your Body: Kabbalah, Mindfulness and Embodied Spiritual Practice* (GodinYourBody, 2007), 176–177.

touched the edge [*kanaph*] of his cloak, and immediately *her hemorrhaging* stopped. (Luke 8:43–44)

This woman had endured twelve years of ceaseless hemorrhage. As a Jew, she was likely aware of the Messianic prophecy regarding the healing power of the "wings" of his garment from Malachi 4:2. With unwavering determination, she forged her path through the throng around Jesus. She then stood in close proximity behind Him, casting a quick, cautious glance around.

Even amidst the pressing crowd, each person was cautious not to touch Jesus' *tzitzit* out of dignity and respect. However, in a moment of bold and audacious desperation, she touched His *tzitzit*. The relentless and crippling torrent of her blood affliction, akin to a tempest in full fury, came to a sudden halt. The Messianic prophecy from Malachi 4:2 had indeed come alive.

> And Jesus said, "Who *is* the one who touched me?" And *when they* all denied *it*, Peter said, "Master, the crowds are pressing you hard and crowding *you*!" But Jesus said, "Someone touched me, because I know power has gone out from me." And *when* the woman saw that she did not escape notice, she came trembling and falling down before him. In the presence of all the people, she told for what reason she had touched him, and that she was healed immediately. And he said to her, "Daughter, your faith has saved you. Go in peace." (Luke 8:45–48)

> When a woman discharges a body fluid *consisting* of her blood *for* many days, *but* not at the time of her menstruation, or when she discharges in addition to her menstruation, all the days of her unclean body fluid discharge she shall become unclean as *in* the days of her menstruation. (Lev. 15:25)

Jesus turned around and asked who had touched His clothing, revealing He felt the healing power surge forth from Him through the touch (Luke 8:46). The woman came forward, trembling with fear that she might be punished; she was not supposed to touch anyone, as she was unclean according to Leviticus 15:25. The Mosaic Law dictated that any object or person coming into contact with an individual deemed unclean would also become unclean (Num. 19:22).

When this woman pressed through the crowd, her body inadvertently brushed against other individuals. To make things even more dire, she even touched the *tzitzit* of Jesus. This could have resulted in the crowd's vehement condemnation, escalating to the peril of her getting stoned to death. She was fearful that Jesus might punish her for touching Him and others while in an unclean state, thereby violating the Mosaic Law.

Instead, Jesus embraced her as His own daughter, shielding her from condemnation, retribution, or punishment. This acknowledgment served as a public declaration of her acceptance as a cherished member of the chosen people of God. This act of redeeming kindness by Jesus was foreshadowed by Boaz, a type of Christ. His immediate reaction to Ruth's bold approach under cover of night was also to call her "my daughter" (Ruth 3:10). Both Ruth, an outsider in a foreign land, and the unnamed woman, marked as unclean due to ceaseless hemorrhaging, were ostracized by society, sharing in their struggles as social outcasts. Both women received acceptance and hope against all odds.

Jesus proclaimed the unnamed woman as cleansed and whole, bestowing upon her the profound honor of serving as a living testament to the fulfillment of the Messianic prophecy. The fact that the woman was suffering for *twelve* years is significant. The number twelve in Judaism symbolizes wholeness and completion.[5] Additionally, Jesus restored her life-giving capacity, an element that was considered essential for women in the first-century Jewish community.

---

5 Brian K. Blount, *Revelation: A Commentary* (Louisville: Presbyterian Publishing, 2013), 387.

The ABC (Abstract to Brick Concrete)

Child (Son, Daughter)—General Definition:[6]

- A son or daughter of human parents; descendent; product, result.

Child (Son, Daughter)—Biblical Definition:

- An individual who, through faith, regardless of social standing, past sins, or worldly labels, is embraced by God's love and grace, becoming a cherished member of His divine family.

The FAST (Focused, Actionable Steps to Take)

Extend a helping hand to those society has overlooked and neglected, recognizing them as our beloved brothers and sisters in Christ. Assist them in reintegrating into our community. Connect with social outcasts and marginalized individuals in meaningful ways, offering not just practical help but also the love and hope of Christ.

Example 1: Becky volunteers with programs that assist formerly incarcerated Christians in rejoining society. She helps them with job training, offers counseling, and shares her faith, guiding them to a fresh start in the context of God's love and forgiveness.

Example 2: Jaime, a professional baker, visits a local Christian orphanage monthly, bringing freshly baked pastries to express Christ's love and compassion. Her commitment brings comfort and warmth to the children, serving up more than just treats but also kindness and care.

Example 3: In the First Baptist Church community, several individuals have come together to offer financial support to local

---

6 "Child," Merriam-Webster.com, accessed October 23, 2023, https://www.merriam-webster.com.

addiction recovery programs. They also open their church to host support group meetings. Additionally, they extend invitations for them to join their church services.

4

A Legacy of Faithfulness —Manasseh

> *Hezekiah became king when he* was *twenty-five years old, and he reigned twenty-nine years in Jerusalem. The name of his mother* was *Abijah, the daughter of Zechariah. And he did that which was right in the eyes of Yahweh, according to all that David his father had done. . . .*
>
> *Hezekiah slept with his ancestors, and they buried him in the upper* part *of the burial sites of the descendants of David. All Judah and the inhabitants of Jerusalem did him honor at his death. And Manasseh, his son, became king in his place.*
>
> Second Chronicles 29:1–2; 32:33

KING MANASSEH of Judah was raised in a devout family, where the generation before him faithfully served and worshipped God. His father, Hezekiah, was exemplary in his faithfulness, and his mother, Hephzibah, was the beloved daughter of the prophet Isaiah.[1] After his father's passing, Manasseh rose to the

---
1 Mark Biltz, *Decoding the Prophet Jeremiah: What an Ancient Prophet Says about Today* (Lake Mary, FL: Charisma House, 2020), 14.

throne at the age of twelve. He forsook the righteous path of his upbringing, casting aside its devout teachings. He traversed the treacherous path of wickedness, marked by abhorrent practices like child sacrifice, idolatrous worship, unjust rule, and the cruel oppression of the vulnerable. In addition, he was known for the persecution of Yahweh's prophets, engagement in witchcraft, astrology, necromancy, and fortune-telling.

> Yahweh brought the commanders of the army of the king of Assyria upon them, and they took Manasseh captive with hooks. They bound him with bronze fetters and brought him to Babylon. And when he was in distress he entreated Yahweh his God and greatly humbled himself before the God of his ancestors and prayed to Him. And God responded to him and heard his plea and let him return to Jerusalem to his kingdom. And Manasseh knew that Yahweh was God. (2 Chron. 33:11–13)

King Manasseh was wicked for thirty-five relentless years, and as a consequence, Yahweh allowed him to fall into the hands of his enemies for all his inequities, evildoings, and wickedness. The nation of Assyria launched an attack on Judah, capturing and imprisoning its king, Manasseh. The Assyrians took Manasseh away to the Babylonian dungeon.

In that dim and forsaken place, he grappled with the harsh realities of his captivity for what must have felt like a never-ending year. King Manasseh sat there, deprived of the luxuries of his throne, with a broken spirit and his pride shattered. Yet, within the depths of his isolation and despair, something remarkable happened. In the solitude of that dungeon, where his very existence hung by a thread, he remembered the God Yahweh his parents had faithfully served. Overwhelmed with remorse, he repented wholeheartedly, his cries for forgiveness echoing off the cold stone walls. In His boundless compassion and mercy, God heard his desperate plea. Manasseh, the humbled king who had tasted the bitter cup of suffering, was forgiven and granted a remarkable second chance. He was allowed to return to his homeland, Judah, where he once more ruled as a mighty king for twenty years.

> He removed the foreign gods and the carved image from the house of Yahweh and all the altars which he built on the mountain of the house of Yahweh and in Jerusalem, and he threw them outside the city. And he restored the altar of Yahweh and offered sacrifices of peace offerings and thank offerings upon it. And he commanded Judah to serve Yahweh, the God of Israel. (2 Chron. 33:15–16)

King Manasseh's sincere repentance marked a pivotal moment, not only on a personal level but also on a national scale. Inspired by divine intervention, he led the entire nation of Judah in purging idolatry from God's house and restoring pure worship for Yahweh as the one and only God. Swiftly, they banished the idols, reinstating Yahweh's sacred altar. With offerings of peace and gratitude, they reclaimed their faith. This commitment endured for the next two decades until Manasseh's passing, a testament to the lasting transformation.

This transformation was possible because of the pious influence of Manasseh's parents, particularly his father, Hezekiah. The devout upbringing and exemplary role models in his life laid the foundation for this change. Hezekiah's steadfast devotion to Yahweh served as a guiding light for Manasseh. He followed in his father's footsteps, both in his personal life and in ruling the kingdom of Judah, to ensure that they remained faithful to God.

The enduring change following repentance highlights the significance of a righteous upbringing and the presence of virtuous role models. It was the values instilled in Manasseh by his parents that allowed him to not only find redemption personally but also to lead Judah on the path of unwavering faithfulness to God. It serves as a powerful testament to the impact of a pious family environment and the positive influence of parents as role models in shaping the destiny of nations.

The ABC (Abstract to Brick Concrete)

Piety—General Definition:[2]
- Showing reverence for deity and devotion to divine worship; marked by conspicuous religiosity; sacred as distinct from the profane or secular.

Piety—Biblical Definition:
- Possessing a knowledge and understanding of God, which can guide the individual to lead a righteous life.

Legacy—General Definition:[3]
- A gift by will especially of money or other personal property; something transmitted by or received from an ancestor or predecessor or from the past.

Legacy—Biblical Definition:
- An enduring impact and example set by devoted Christians, including their steadfast faith, commitment to Christian principles, and their practical application in daily life.

The FAST (Focused, Actionable Steps to Take)

1. Make an effort to gain knowledge and an understanding of God, as this will help you differentiate between what's good and what's not. This will enable you to align your actions with His will and principles.

   Example: Seth, a business owner, is a strong believer who never misses a Sunday service. On leaving work one evening,

---

[2] "Piety," Merriam-Webster.com, accessed October 23, 2023, https://www.merriam-webster.com.

[3] "Legacy," Merriam-Webster.com, accessed October 23, 2023, https://www.merriam-webster.com.

A Legacy of Faithfulness—Manasseh 41

he discovered the flower bed in front of the building in disarray and initially suspected the groundskeeper, Chuck, as the one responsible. He was on the verge of firing Chuck in his anger. However, recalling the teachings from his Sunday service about the importance of being "quick to hear, slow to speak, slow to anger" (James 1:19–20), Seth decided to approach Chuck to discuss the situation. To Seth's surprise, Chuck revealed that he had caught a mole responsible for the damage and even volunteered to work an extra shift to repair it at no additional cost.

2. Parents should set an example for their children by faithfully serving God. They should create an environment where their children can practice a devout and pious way of life, which includes daily Scripture study, prayer, and worship. This solid foundation will enable their children to live a life in communion with God. Even if they stray from their faith, they will know how to return and live faithfully.

Example: Isaac and Veronica are steadfast Christians, firmly rooted in their faith. Their daughters, Amanda and Lillian, faithfully engage in evening Scripture study, prayer, and worship alongside their parents. As a family, they wholeheartedly embrace the teachings of Christ in their daily lives. This enduring legacy continues beyond their lifetimes, shining as a guiding light for their daughters and the generations to come.

5

A Legacy of Impiety—Ahab

But Omri did evil in the eyes of Yahweh more than all who were before him. He went in all the way of Jeroboam the son of Nebat and in his sins that he caused Israel to sin by provoking Yahweh the God of Israel with their idols.

First Kings 16:25–26

Now Ahab son of Omri became king over Israel in the thirty-eighth year of Asa king of Judah. Ahab son of Omri reigned over Israel in Samaria twenty-two years. But Ahab son of Omri did evil in the eyes of Yahweh more than all who were before him. **If it wasn't enough that he went** *after the sins of Jeroboam the son of Nebat, he also took as wife Jezebel the daughter of Ethbaal the king of the Sidonians. He went and served Baal and bowed down to him. He built an altar to Baal in the house of Baal which he had built in Samaria.*

First Kings 16:29–32

KING AHAB OF Israel was raised in a household of idolatry, with his father, King Omri, known for doing "evil in the eyes of Yahweh more than all who were before him" (1 Kings 16:25). Ahab's marriage to Jezebel, an ardent idol worshipper, further immersed him in this ungodly environment. Throughout his upbringing and life, he bore witness to his family's involvement in various sinful and wicked practices to the extent that he knew no other way of living.

Ahab continued to live in a wicked and evil way, his heart steeped in darkness, until he committed the heinous act of murdering an innocent man to illegitimately seize his land. It was in this abyss of moral decay that Yahweh sent a divine message, forewarning Ahab of his impending death—a death that would be both publicly humiliating and dishonorable, a reckoning for his transgressions.

> Thus says Yahweh: "Have you committed murder and also taken possession? . . . In the place where the dogs licked the blood of Naboth, the dogs will also lick your blood." (1 Kings 21:19)
>
> When Ahab heard these words, he tore his clothes and put sackcloth over his flesh, fasted, lay in the sackcloth, and went about dejectedly. Then the word of Yahweh came to Elijah the Tishbite, saying, "Have you seen how Ahab has humbled himself before me? Because he has humbled himself before me, I will not bring disaster in his days. I will bring the disaster to his house in the days of his son." (21:27–29)

Confronted by God's foreboding warning, King Ahab humbled himself in repentance for all the evil deeds, idolatry, wickedness, and iniquities. In response, God decided to delay the impending judgment on these transgressions to the next generation.

His repentance had not stirred a single ripple of transformation in the way he conducted his life or ruled the nation of Israel. His upbringing in the wicked atmosphere of the house of Omri was decidedly secular; no one had shown or taught him how to live a life faithful to Yahweh. He had no strong, devout role model in his immediate circle, no foundation of faith, and no moral compass to distinguish between right and wrong—and yet, he repented at the preaching of Elijah! Soon afterward, however, Ahab descended into a spiral of sinful wickedness and evil deeds. His very essence was steeped in the dark waters of sin, and he was oblivious to any other way of existence.

> Then the king [Ahab] said to him [Micaiah], "How many times must I make you swear that you shall not tell me *anything* but the truth in the name of Yahweh?" So he said, "I saw all of Israel scattering to the mountains, like the sheep without a shepherd. Yahweh also said, 'There are no masters for these, let them return in peace, each to his house.'" Then the king of Israel said to Jehoshaphat, "Did I not say to you that he would not prophesy good concerning me, but disaster?" . . .
>
> The king of Israel said, "Take Micaiah and return him to Amon the commander of the city and to Jehoash the son of the king; and say, 'Thus says the king: "Put this *fellow in* the house of imprisonment and feed him reduced rations of food and water until I come in peace."'" (1 Kings 22:16–18, 26–27)

Three years had passed since his profound repentance, yet King Ahab remained entrenched in his unrelenting wickedness. The prophet Micaiah foretold that Israel would not emerge victorious in its battle against the Arameans at Ramoth in Gilead. Enraged by the divine message delivered by the prophet, Ahab persisted in going to battle, hoping to defy the sacred revelation and win. However, the revelation proved true, and Ahab met his demise in the battle.

Ahab's struggle to live a virtuous life after repentance stems, in part, from the lack of a role model in his life, leaving him without guidance in serving and worshipping Yahweh. This legacy of impiety left him without guiding principles to distinguish right from wrong. This tragedy highlights the significance of environmental influence from early life on the spiritual connection with God.

The ABC (Abstract to Brick Concrete)

Impiety—General Definition:[1]

- Lacking in reverence or proper respect for God.

Impiety—Biblical Definition:

- Lacking true knowledge and understanding of God, often leading individuals to live in evil and wicked ways.

The FAST (Focused, Actionable Steps to Take)

1. Make an effort to gain the knowledge and understanding of God, as this will help you discern between good and evil, giving you a choice to make the right choices in life.

    Example: Harry attends Sunday service at his church every week. Through consistent exposure to biblical teachings, the principle of justice became ingrained within him. He is guided by the biblical standards in his role as a city councilor. He develops policies to promote social justice and care for the marginalized and neglected in the community.

2. Parents should create an environment where their children can learn the Scriptures and develop the wisdom to discern between good and evil. Without this foundation, they will face significant spiritual hurdles to come to faith and lead a righteous life.

    Example: Marcus and Hannah had been more focused on their wealth and careers, somewhat detached from God and His principles. However, as their daughter Sally grew up, they offered her the option to attend church to learn about God. Since then, Sally has been actively participating in church activities and immersing herself in the study of divine principles.

---

1 "Impiety," Merriam-Webster.com, accessed October 23, 2023, https://www.merriam-webster.com.

6

Highways to Zion

How lovely are *your dwelling places, O Yahweh of hosts! My soul longs and even fails for the courtyards of Yahweh. My heart and flesh sing for joy to the living God. Even a bird finds a home, and a swallow a nest for herself, where she may lay her young, near your altars, O Yahweh of hosts, my king and my God. Blessed* are *those who dwell in your house; they can ever praise you.* **Selah**

Psalm 84:1–4

PSALM 84 ILLUSTRATES a man's heartfelt longing to dwell in the presence of God. This desire transcends any material aspirations, such as seeking wealth, fertility, health, or longevity, as it solely revolves around the profound yearning for a close relationship with Him. The psalmist even mentions how a bird found a blessing in nesting near the altars, underscoring that those in the house of worship are truly blessed as they can ever praise Him. The purity and divine focus of this worship are refreshing, especially in this generation often dominated by the prosperity gospel.

> Blessed *is* the man whose strength *is* in you;
> in their heart *are the* highways *to Zion*.
> Passing through the Valley of Baca,

they make it a spring.
The early rain covers *it with* blessings as well.
They go from strength to strength,
until each appears before God in Zion.
(Ps. 84:5–7)

In the ancient days of the Old Testament, devout followers of Yahweh often embarked on pilgrimages to the holy Temple in Zion. Their hearts were filled with a continuous yearning to return to the house of God as they gazed upon the highways to Zion. With this deep reverence and longing, the psalmist wrote of the highways to Zion etched in their hearts.

In due course, Jesus Christ came and cleansed our sins with His blood, making us clean and holy. Through the blood of Christ, we gained the privilege to stand before God in a state of grace and forgiveness. Christ then sent the Holy Spirit to dwell within us, transforming us into the house of God (1 Cor. 3:16). Now God resides within our hearts, akin to His presence in the holy Temple of Zion. Just as ancient pilgrims journeyed the highways to Zion to seek him, Christ has become the pathway through which we enter the presence of our heavenly Father.

The psalmist praises God for bestowing renewed strength upon those who place their trust solely in Him rather than in humankind. He goes on to describe how the pilgrims, with their renewed strength, transformed the Valley of Baca into a spring. The Hebrew word *Baca* means "balsam trees," which are known to thrive in arid regions and exude resin, like tears. Balsam trees, therefore, have long been associated with weeping or affliction.[1]

The Valley of Baca is likely a metaphorical expression for any desolate region invigorated by the passage of many pilgrims. They received overflowing strength, exceeding their own needs. They then used the excess to have a positive influence on their surroundings.

---
1 Willem A. Van Gemeren, *Expositor's Bible Commentary: Psalms* (Grand Rapids: Zondervan, 2008), 636.

In a similar vein, Christ has given us overflowing love, grace, and forgiveness. It is incumbent upon us to share the precious gifts from Christ with the people we encounter in our journey through life.

> Behold, Yahweh *was* standing beside him, and he said, "I *am* Yahweh, the God of Abraham your father, and the God of Isaac. The ground on which you *were* sleeping I will give to you and to your descendants. Your descendants shall be like the dust of the earth, and you will spread out to the west, and to the east, and to the north and to the south. All the families of the earth will be blessed through you and through your descendants. Now behold, I *am* with you, and I will keep you wherever you go. I will bring you to this land, for I will not leave you until I have done what I have promised to you." (Gen. 28:13–15)

In this covenant, God committed to protect, restore, and bring forth blessings to all nations through Jacob's lineage. In his most troubled days, the psalmist clings to the Covenant God, steadfastly awaiting His deliverance.

> O Yahweh, God of hosts, hear my prayer;
> give ear, O God of Jacob. *Selah*
> Look at our shield, O God,
> and have regard for the face of your anointed one.
> Because better is a day in your courtyards
> than a thousand *elsewhere*.
> I would rather be at the threshold of the house of my God
> than to dwell in *the* tents of wickedness.
> Because Yahweh God *is* a sun and a shield;
> Yahweh gives grace and honor.
> He does not withhold good from those who walk blamelessly.
> O Yahweh *of* hosts,
> blessed *is the* man who trusts you.
>
> (Ps. 84:8–12)

In this prayer, Yahweh is referred to as the God of Jacob because of the covenant He made with the patriarch Jacob. This covenant was passed down to Jacob's descendants, which includes this psalmist.

The writer strongly invokes the characteristics of Yahweh. He portrays Him as the Sun radiating its light of life with "grace" and glory ("honor"). He also refers to Him as the Defender ("shield"), highlighting His just ("He does not withhold good from those who walk blamelessly.") and faithful ("blessed is the man who trusts you.") nature. He also addresses Him as the God of hosts, highlighting His sovereignty.

The ABC (Abstract to Brick Concrete)

Temple—General Definition:[2]

- A building for religious practice.

Temple—Biblical Definition:

- Each believer in whom God resides; relying on one's relationship with God rather than physical places.

The FAST (Focused, Actionable Steps to Take)

Practice mutual respect, service, and compassion in your interactions with others in your faith community. Offer support and help to those in need.

Example 1: Embracing the idea of viewing fellow Christians as temples of God has brought significant benefits to the Riverside Church community. Many members have found renewed purpose and fulfillment through practicing mutual respect and service. This shift has strengthened relationships, deepening understanding, compassion, and unity among them. They now

---

[2] "Temple," Merriam-Webster.com, accessed October 23, 2023, https://www.merriam-webster.com.

share a willingness to support one another, particularly in times of need. This change has enriched their spiritual lives and created an inviting atmosphere where everyone feels valued and supported. As a result, the Riverside Church has become a place of solace, growth, and unwavering fellowship, guided by the belief that God resides within each of them.

Example 2: Melanie offers words of encouragement and affirmation to her fellow Christians. Her kind words and unwavering support serve as a source of strength, fortifying the faith of those around her.

7

From the Tax Ladder to the Heavenly Elevator— Zacchaeus

He entered and *traveled through Jericho. And* there was *a man* named *Zacchaeus, and he* was *a chief tax collector, and he* was *rich. And he was seeking to see Jesus—who he was—and he was not able to as a result of the crowd, because he was short in stature.*

Luke 19:1–3

Indeed, any man in whom is a physical defect shall not come near: a blind man or lame or disfigured or deformed, or a man in whom is a broken foot or a broken hand, or a hunchback or a dwarf, or a spot in his eye or a skin disorder or a skin eruption or a crushed testicle.

Leviticus 21:18–20

JESUS WAS PASSING through Jericho with his disciples one day on his way to Jerusalem for the Great Passover. Jericho was a prosperous city with considerable political influence throughout the nation. Within this opulent city, Zacchaeus, the chief tax collector, oversaw the division of taxation. His role, akin to a tax commissioner today, earned him the disdain of fellow Jews. This animosity stemmed from the perception that tax collectors for the Roman Empire were traitors to the Jewish nation. Their corrupt tax practices garnered them notoriety as extortionists and thieves, further plummeting their social standing to the lowest of lows.[1] Subsequently, tax collectors were excommunicated from the synagogues for both social and religious reasons; it was the customary and devastating consequence of their profession.[2]

The Gospels reflect this social stigma, often associating tax collectors with sinners, Gentiles, and prostitutes (Matt. 18:17; 21:31; Luke 15:1). Furthermore, in the social and religious context of that era, riches were not always viewed as a mark of virtue; rather, wealth often carried a neutral or even negative connotation (Prov. 11:4; 15:16; 22:1–2; 28:6; Isa. 5:8).

In Luke 19:3, the Greek word used for "short" is *mikros*, which can be translated as "pathological dwarfism."[3] This interpretation gains credibility because Luke, who described him using this term, was a physician. His need to climb a tall tree because of his short stature to see Jesus further supports the idea that he indeed suffered from dwarfism. The Greek word *mikros* finds its

---

1 James S. Jeffers, *The Greco-Roman World of the New Testament Era: Exploring the Background of Early Christianity* (Downers Grove, IL: Inter-Varsity Press, 1999), 146.

2 R.T. France and David Wenham, *Gospel Perspectives, Volume 3: Studies in Midrash and Historiography* (Eugene, OR: Wipf and Stock, 2003), 207.

3 Amos Yong, "Zacchaeus: Short and Un-Seen," in *Christian Reflection: A Series in Faith and Ethics Disability* , ed. Robert B. Kruschwitz (Waco, TX: The Center for Christian Ethics at Baylor University, 2012), 11–17.

equivalence in the Hebrew term *daq*.[4] In Leviticus 21:18–20, dwarfism (*daq*) is listed among the twelve physical blemishes, alongside leprosy and blindness, which render individuals ineligible for priestly service.

Zacchaeus, burdened by a religiously stigmatized disability, his role as chief tax collector, and his wealth, became a social leper. He bore the weight of public odium in the bustling streets of Jericho. He endured not only disdain and ridicule but also the collective judgment of his community. The townspeople held him in contempt, considering him unworthy of their acceptance. He was not just an outsider; he was the embodiment of what they loathed.

Zacchaeus was outwardly a wealthy man, but within, he felt impoverished, tormented by loneliness, isolation, and suffering from the disdain and loathing that his community directed toward him. As time passed, his suffering only intensified, and he could not find any relief. As he learned of the imminent arrival of Jesus, the Miracle Healer renowned for even raising the dead, Zacchaeus clung to this last glimmer of hope for healing.

> He ran on ahead *and* climbed up into a sycamore tree so that he could see him, because he was going to go through *that way*. When he came to the place, Jesus looked up *and* said to him, "Zacchaeus, come down quickly, because it is necessary *for* me to stay at your house today!" He came down quickly and welcomed him joyfully. (Luke 19:4–6)

As the tree came into view, Zacchaeus ran toward it and quickly climbed up in his eagerness to see Jesus. At that moment, Jesus showed up, surrounded by nearly 5,000 people in the crowd. To his astonishment, Jesus walked directly to the tree where Zacchaeus clung and tenderly called him by name,

---

4 Muhammad Wolfgang G.A. Schmidt, *A Hebrew-English Reference Manual To The Hebrew Text Of The Old Testament* (Hamburg, Germany: disserta Verlag, 2017), 142.

his voice filled with love and compassion. What followed was equally unexpected as Jesus invited himself to Zacchaeus' mansion. Overjoyed, his heart brimming with newfound hope, he led Jesus to his mansion. Jesus, the Giver of life, came to rescue Zacchaeus from the tree, thus moving him from a life of spiritual death to a new life.

> *When they* saw *it*, they all began to complain, saying, "He has gone in to find lodging with a man who is a sinner!" Zacchaeus stopped *and* said to the Lord, "Behold, half of my possessions, Lord, I am giving to the poor, and if I have extorted anything from anyone, I am paying *it* back four times *as much*!" (Luke 19:7–8)

The Greek word used for "all" in 19:7 is *pantes*, which is a word of inclusion, referring to the whole community.[5] Zacchaeus was condemned as a sinner and outcast, rejected not only by the Pharisees but by the entire society, denying his rights as a Jew and his place among the people of God. As Jesus and Zacchaeus walked to the house, the people of Jericho began to grumble about Jesus staying with him, such an unforgivable sinner.

Jesus' companionship with Zacchaeus greatly tarnished His reputation. The grace of Jesus especially rattled the religious and social leaders, leaving them scandalized. The disparaging remarks toward Jesus deeply troubled Zacchaeus. He recognized the inherent conflict in attempting to simultaneously pursue Jesus and cling to his worldly riches (Matt. 6:24). This pivotal moment forced him to make a resolute decision to follow Jesus and abandon the pursuit of material affluence. He boldly proclaimed his resolve to give half his possessions to the poor and to make fourfold restitution to anyone he had extorted. It was more than a mere act of charity; it was a public declaration of his profound transformation into a follower of Christ.

---

5 Dorothy Kelley Patterson and Rhonda Harrington Kelley, *Women's Evangelical Commentary: New Testament* (Nashville: B&H Publishing Group, 2011), 522.

Jesus said to him, "Today salvation has come to this house, because he too is a son of Abraham. For the Son of Man came to seek and to save those who are lost." (Luke 19:9–10)

> Blessed *are* the poor in spirit,
> because theirs is the kingdom of heaven.
> (Matt. 5:3)

Before anyone in the crowd had the chance to cast Zacchaeus aside in general contempt, Jesus stepped forward to bestow His grace, an unmerited gift, upon the wretched outcast in full view of the public. Zacchaeus did not attain salvation based on his words or actions. Instead, the gift of the kingdom of heaven was graciously bestowed upon him, entirely undeserved. Jesus granted him the kingdom of heaven because of this materially wealthy man's spiritual poverty. He replenished Zacchaeus' spirit with love, compassion, and hope. Then, Jesus revealed that He, the Son of Man, had come to seek and save Zacchaeus, who was among the lost. Zacchaeus had been lost in the pursuit of material possessions, and yet, none of the religious leaders had ventured to bring him back. No one had gone in search of him. Jesus came to seek and save those who were marginalized. In this act of redemption, Jesus also bestowed upon him the title of "son of Abraham," thereby restoring him into the community for the people of God.

Before anyone in the crowd could condemn Zacchaeus, Jesus stepped forward to affirm his status as a son of Abraham. This designation carried significant meaning, as descendants of Abraham were heirs to the divine covenants that promised protection, restoration, and blessings to all nations through them. In acknowledging Zacchaeus as a son of Abraham, Jesus, the covenant God, was recognizing his rightful place within the Jewish community and expressing His commitment to fulfill these promises to Zacchaeus.

Despite his immense material wealth, he had a profound spiritual poverty. This spiritual poverty manifested as a lack of inner peace, joy, hope, love, and compassion. His pursuit of material wealth and worldly gain had left him empty in the aspects of life that truly matter. When Zacchaeus embraced Jesus as his Savior, he experienced a profound transformation akin to receiving the kingdom of heaven in his life. In this context, the "kingdom of heaven" represents salvation and all the spiritual blessings that come with it. His inner change marked the end of his spiritual poverty and brought fulfillment and joy through his newfound relationship with God.

The ABC (Abstract to Brick Concrete)

Salvation—General Definition:[6]
- Deliverance from the power and effects of sin; liberation from ignorance or illusion; preservation from death or failure; deliverance from danger or difficulty.

Salvation—Biblical Definition
- Divine transformation of an individual's life, where through faith, they are reconciled with God and empowered to live a new, Christ-centered existence; shifting one's focus from worldly pursuits to a deep commitment to knowing, serving, and following Christ in their thoughts, actions, and relationships.

The FAST (Focused, Actionable Steps to Take)

Replace tempting habits with activities that align with your faith and support a Christ-centered way of living. Identify those habits that lead you away from Christ's teachings, and consciously choose alternatives that bring you closer to Him.

---

6 "Salvation," Merriam-Webster.com, accessed October 23, 2023, https://www.merriam-webster.com.

Example 1: Marcus used to listen to rock-and-roll music with explicit lyrics while commuting to and from work, often singing along with profanity. To make his daily routine more Christ-centered, he decided to switch to listening to Christian music during his commutes. This change allowed him to use his travel time for worship and reflection.

Example 2: Nancy struggled with alcohol addiction but realized it wasn't helping her anxiety. So, she switched to prayer, giving all her worries to God instead. This shift allowed her to manage her anxiety in a healthier way and grow in her faith.

A Quote to Ponder

> *Pride loves to climb up, not as Zacchaeus,*
> *to see Christ, but to be seen himself.*
>
> William Gurnall[7]

---

7 William Gurnall, *The Christian in Complete Armour* (London: William Tegg, 1862), 139.

8

Life, Death, and Re-Nain-ssance

It happened that on the next day *he went to a town called Nain, and his disciples and a large crowd went with him. And as he approached the gate of the town, behold, a man who had died was being carried out, his mother's only son, and she was a widow. And a large crowd from the town was with her.*

Luke 7:11–12

FROM THE SYNOPTIC Gospels, we learn that Jesus chose the city of Capernaum in the region of Galilee as the focal point for His divine ministry.[1] Capernaum, a city of commerce with nearly 3,000 inhabitants, witnessed the bustling traffic of a diverse array of people passing through its streets. In stark contrast, Nain, situated approximately twenty-five miles (forty kilometers) from Capernaum, was a destitute farming village. It housed a meager population of 100–120

---

1 Titus M. Kennedy, *Excavating the Evidence for Jesus* (Eugene, OR: Harvest House, 2022), 102–103.

men residing within fewer than thirty-five houses.[2] Access to this impoverished hamlet was granted only through a rugged, unpaved path that bore the weight of neglect. Given the deplored state of the road, walking from Capernaum to Nain would have been an arduous expedition, spanning ten to twelve hours or more.

In Luke 7, we find Jesus leaving the city of Capernaum with a large crowd trailing behind him. After a grueling half-day of walking, they arrived at the destitute hamlet, Nain. Upon their arrival, an unanticipated scene unfolded before them—a funeral procession coming out of the village. The heaviness of the moment was palpable as it became evident that they were bearing the lifeless body of a young man. They were heading to a nearby cemetery for his burial. Walking alongside was the young man's grieving mother, dressed in the heavy shroud of widow's attire. Her chest heaved with the weight of an unbearable loss, each breath a struggle to find solace in a world that had become unrecognizable. Overwhelmed by the depths of her sorrow, she was rendered speechless, unable to utter a single word.

> *When* the Lord saw her, he had compassion for her and said to her, "Do not weep!" He came up *and* touched the bier, and those who were carrying *it* stopped. He said, "Young man, I say to you, get up!" And the dead man sat up and began to speak, and he gave him to his mother. (7:13–15)

> The one who touches a corpse of *any person* will be unclean for seven days. . . . Anything that the unclean *person* touches will be unclean, and the person who touches *it* will be unclean until the evening. (Num. 19:11, 22)

> When a person touches anything unclean, *whether* human uncleanness or an unclean animal or any unclean detestable thing, and he eats from the meat of the fellowship offerings'

---

2 Eric Mills, *Census of Palestine 1931*, Vol. I (Alexandria, Egypt: Whitehead Morris Ltd., 1933), 75.

sacrifice, which *is* for Yahweh, then that person shall be cut off from his people. (Lev. 7:21)

He [Jesus] summoned the twelve and began to send them out two *by* two, and gave them authority over the unclean spirits. (Mark 6:7)

Summoning his twelve disciples, he [Jesus] gave them authority over unclean spirits, so that they could expel *them* and could heal every disease and every sickness. (Matt. 10:1)

As Jesus gazed into her eyes, He saw unfathomable sorrow and emptiness reflected within them. He felt a profound sympathy for the unbearable sadness, despair, and devastation dwelling in the depths of her being. Without hesitation, He approached her directly, and their eyes met in a meaningful connection. At that moment, she looked upon this stranger, sensing that His eyes saw through her as if He understood every ounce of her suffering. With a gentle and compassionate voice, Jesus spoke to her, saying, "Do not weep." Little did she know that He had journeyed here for half a day, not to add to her sorrow but to bring laughter out of her mourning.

Jesus touched the bier of her son's coffin, an item considered unclean under the Mosaic Law, which prohibited contact with anything impure due to the belief that uncleanness would spread. The onlookers, shocked by the sight of Jesus touching the unclean, stared in disbelief at the unfolding scene. It merits attention that Jesus possessed authority over unclean spirits, a power He also bestowed upon His disciples (Mark 6:7; Matt. 10:1). At His command, life returned to the body. His authority over the dominion of death and unclean spirits left the crowds in awe. Jesus then offered the revived young man to his mother, who, now filled with an overwhelming joy, couldn't contain her laughter. This miraculous turnaround is a characteristic of God portrayed consistently throughout the Scriptures (Ps. 30:11; Jer. 31:13; Isa. 61:3).

There are individuals whose hearts are so shattered that they become utterly speechless, unable to find the words to articulate their needs or to reach out for help. In these moments, God's boundless grace extends to deliver them, even when they are unable to call out for His help, for He knows the depth of suffering beneath their silence. The unrequested act of redemption depicted in Luke 7:11–17 is a demonstration of God's transcendent grace.

> Fear seized *them* all, and they began to glorify God, saying, "A great prophet has appeared among us!" and "God has visited to help his people!" And this report about him went out in the whole of Judea and in all the surrounding region. (7:16–17)

The crowd was filled with fear upon realizing they were in the presence of God. This holy terror arises when our own transgressions and imperfections are laid bare before God, who is holy and flawless. This fear of God led them to repent and glorify God. This revival didn't confine itself to Judah alone but extended its influence to all the surrounding nations.

The ABC (Abstract to Brick Concrete)

Uncleanness—General Definition:[3]

- Dirty; filthy; morally or spiritually impure; infected with a harmful supernatural contagion.

Uncleanness—Biblical Definition

- Possessing a trait that God declared as ceremonially impure in the Old Testament; twisted by sinful individuals, religious teachers, and society into a reason to cruelly stigmatize, thus linked with pervasive bias and prejudice, resulting in heightened susceptibility to exclusion,

---

[3] "Uncleanness," Merriam-Webster.com, accessed October 23, 2023, https://www.merriam-webster.com.

discrimination, and mistreatment; the unclean were wrongly seen as "being" their uncleanness and having an impure identity; by the grace of God, the teachings of Christ redefined "uncleanness" as an opportunity for compassion, healing, and breaking down societal barriers.

The FAST (Focused, Actionable Steps to Take)

Offer assistance, compassion, and acceptance to those who are marginalized or often regarded as outcasts in our daily interactions.

Example: Every month, Chad visits the prison to lead Bible study sessions for the inmates, fostering an environment of spiritual growth and reflection. Through his actions and words, Chad conveys the profound love and kindness taught by Christ, creating a sense of hope, support, and understanding among the incarcerated individuals. His commitment to the inmates serves as a testament to the transformative power of faith and compassion, making a positive impact on the lives of those he encounters.

9

Bed and Bible (B&B)—Gaius

The elder, to Gaius the beloved, whom I love in the truth. Dear friend, I pray you may prosper concerning everything and be healthy, just as your soul prospers. For I rejoiced exceedingly when the brothers came and testified to your truth, just as you are walking in the truth. I have no greater joy than this: that I hear my children are walking in the truth.

Third John 1–4

Jesus said to him [Thomas the apostle], *"I am the way, and the truth, and the life. No one comes to the Father except through me."*

John 14:6

THE GREEK WORD *epistole*, meaning a written letter, has given rise to the English term "epistle."[1] In the realm of epistolary communication, we come across the Third Epistle of John

---

1 Eugene E. Carpenter and Philip Wesley Comfort, *Holman Treasury of Key Bible Words* (Nashville: B&H Publishing Group, 2000), 274.

(commonly abbreviated as "3 John"). This letter is a personal message from the apostle John to his fellow Christian, Gaius.

John opens his letter by addressing Gaius as the one he loves in truth. While Third John is among the shortest books in the New Testament, it uses the word "truth" seven times. The Greek term he employed for this word "truth" is *aletheia*, which was also used when Jesus described himself in the Gospel of John 14:6. The original meaning of *aletheia* is "corresponding to reality."[2] Substituting "Christ" for the word "truth" in his message makes the meaning clearer: "the beloved, whom I love in *Christ*," "testified to your *Christ*," and "walking in *Christ*." The word "Christ" may not have been directly used due to the worsening persecution of Christianity at the time this letter was written.

> Dear friend, you act faithfully *in* whatever you do for the brothers, *even though they are strangers*. They have testified *to* your love before the church; you will do well to send them on their way in a manner worthy of God. For they have gone out on behalf of the name, accepting nothing from the pagans. Therefore we ought to support such *people*, so that we become fellow workers with *the* truth. (3 John 5–8)

Substituting "Christ" for "truth" yields the insight that the phrase "fellow workers with the truth" likely alluded to Christians. With this understanding, we can now see that John praised hospitality to traveling gospel preachers as an essential Christian virtue. These preachers declined any financial compensation from unbelievers for spreading the gospel. This unconventional practice demonstrated their commitment to serving God without seeking personal gain. Instead, support for the gospel cause was expected to come from fellow Christians. In this context, Gaius warmly welcomed the missionaries into

---

2 John MacArthur, *1, 2, 3 John and Jude: Established in Truth . . . Marked by Love* (Nashville: Harper Christian Resources, 2016), 86.

his home, where he hosted and supported them and showed genuine kindness.³

In Third John 2, John subtly alluded that Gaius may not have been in the best physical condition, yet spiritually, he had been strong and resilient. With this backdrop, his tireless dedication to serving the traveling ministries becomes even more remarkable. As a result of this hospitality, these missionaries later shared heartfelt commendations about Gaius with John the apostle.

> I wrote something to the church, but Diotrephes, who wants to be first *among* them, does not acknowledge us. Therefore, if I come, I will call attention to *the deeds he is doing*, disparaging us with evil words. Not being content with these, he does not receive the brothers himself, and he hinders those wanting *to do so* and throws *them* out of the church. Dear friend, do not imitate *what is* evil, but *what is* good. The one who does good is of God; the one who does evil has not seen God. (9–11)

Among the church's leaders, it appears that Diotrephes held a prominent position, possibly as an elder. Unfortunately, Diotrephes allowed his pride to lead him to openly defy the authority of apostle John, even resorting to disparaging remarks against him and his teachings. He went as far as excommunicating those who adhered to John's teachings from the church. Instead of promoting unity within the congregation, he relentlessly sought power and dominance. John likely wrote to Gaius about his concerns regarding Diotrephes to caution him not to be swayed by Diotrephes' negative influence. John reassured Gaius that he was on the right path and encouraged him to keep offering hospitality to the messengers of the gospel.

> Demetrius has been testified to by all, even by the truth itself. We also testify to *him*, and you know that our testimony is true. I have many things to write to you, but I do not want to write

---

3 Colin G. Kruse, *The Letters of John* (Grand Rapids: Eerdmans, 2000), 215–223.

to you by means of ink and pen. But I hope to see you right away, and to speak *face to face*. Peace *be* to you. The friends greet you. Greet the friends by name. (3 John 12–15)

John introduced Gaius to a man named Demetrius, whose words and actions align with the teachings of scripture. Demetrius was also steadfastly proven to be righteous, not only to other fellow Christians but also to John himself. It seems that John's message to Gaius was a stern caution, urging him not to follow in the footsteps of Diotrephes by withholding hospitality from Demetrius. The mention of his name at the end of the letter hints at the possibility that he may have served as the bearer of John's epistle to Gaius.

This affectionate letter draws to a close with a personal touch, expressing John's longing to meet them in person. As the sole living apostle at the time, John held the authority to summon Gaius, Diotrephes, and other church leaders. However, in a remarkable display of humility, he committed to embark on a journey to meet them face-to-face. This commitment starkly contrasted with Diotrephes' ambitious actions aimed at elevating himself above others.

The ABC (Abstract to Brick Concrete)

Hospitality—General Definition:[4]

- Hospitable (generous, cordial, friendly) treatment, reception, or disposition, the activity of providing services to guests.

Hospitality—Biblical Definition:

- A way of sharing the burdens of those serving God, recognizing that in doing so, we all work toward a common goal of serving God.

---

4 "Hospitality," Merriam-Webster.com, accessed October 23, 2023, https://www.merriam-webster.com.

The FAST (Focused, Actionable Steps to Take)

Offer your support and assistance to those serving in ministry in ways that are practical and match your abilities. This can be as simple as keeping them in your prayers and sharing words of encouragement.

Example 1: Logan helps missionaries visiting his area by giving them rides to and from the airport.

Example 2: Julie donates 15 percent of her farm produce to missionaries and their families.

10

One Touch of Heaven on the Untouchable

*When **he came down from the mountain, large crowds followed him. And behold, a leper approached** and **worshiped him, saying, "Lord, if you are willing, you are able to make me clean." And extending his hand he touched him, saying, "I am willing, be clean." And immediately his leprosy was cleansed. And Jesus said to him, "See that you tell no one, but go, show yourself to the priest and offer the gift that Moses commanded, for a testimony to them."***

Matthew 8:1–4

As for the person who is afflicted with a skin disease, his garments must be torn and his hair *must* be allowed to hang loosely, and he must cover *his* upper lip, *and he must call out, 'Unclean! Unclean!'* For *all* the *days* during *which the infection* is *on him, he shall be unclean; he must live alone; his dwelling* must be outside the camp.

Leviticus 13:45–46

A MAN, AFFLICTED by the torment of leprosy, suddenly emerged from the woods and began to walk toward Jesus. The large crowd that was surrounding Jesus gasped and hastily moved away from Jesus and the leper. According to the Mosaic Law, the leper, who was unclean, was not supposed to come near the clean. His uncleanness bore the risk of contaminating the purity of the gathered. Despite the threat of getting stoned to death by the crowd, he pressed on until he stood in front of Jesus.

In an act of unyielding desperation, this leper boldly knelt before Christ. Leprosy, an inexorable systemic infection, likely would have severely eroded and deformed his joints.[1] Kneeling, with his disfigured joints, may have led to a fracture of his patella or a tear of his quadriceps tendon.[2] He knelt down, fully knowing he might not be able to rise again.

He said to Jesus, "If you are willing, you can make me clean." Despite his unshakable faith in God's sovereignty, doubt shrouded him, for he knew himself as a wretched sinner, unworthy of redemption. Fully aware that he had no right to healing, this sinner cast himself entirely upon the grace and mercy of Jesus. In response, Jesus stretched forth His hand to touch the untouchable, the leper. As Jesus declared His willingness and commanded cleansing, leprosy immediately left him. With Jesus, a lifetime of despair, a fate echoed by everyone, unraveled in just a second as this astounding transformation took place.

Jesus then kindly advised him to wait until a priest formally declared him clean before telling others of his healing. This was a precaution to avoid the possibility of priests refusing to acknowledge his healing due to their jealousy toward Jesus, which would have prevented this man from getting reintegrated into

---

1 Sandeep Chauhan, Anupam Wakhlu, and Vikas Agarwal, "Arthritis in Leprosy," *Rheumatology* 49 (12): 2237–2242 (2010).

2 Arnold Soren, *Arthritis and Related Affections: Clinic, Pathology, and Treatment* (Berlin, Germany: Springer, 2011), 357.

the community. Jesus sought not just to cure a medical illness but the complete restoration of the individual as a person.

The ABC (Abstract to Brick Concrete)

Desperation—General Definition:[3]

- Loss of hope and surrender to despair, a state of hopelessness leading to rashness.

Desperation—Biblical Definition:

- The driving force that compels one to risk everything in an attempt to seek God's attention, recognizing Him as the sole source of hope, a state of yearning for divine mercy.

The FAST (Focused, Actionable Steps to Take)

1. Share messages of God's love and mercy with those in desperate circumstances. Encourage them to use their desperation as fuel for intense prayer, wholeheartedly seeking Him in their time of need.

   Example: Matthew had a conversation with a friend who had just received a terminal cancer diagnosis. During their talk, he shared the message of the gospel and encouraged his friend to turn to God rather than dwell in despair and hopelessness. Matthew also invited his friend to join him for a Sunday worship service at his church.

2. Follow Christ's example by uplifting and helping the vulnerable, just as He did. Reach out to the marginalized, offering them support, comfort, and renewed hope. Through your actions, show that His message of salvation and grace is very much alive.

---

3 "Desperation," Merriam-Webster.com, accessed October 23, 2023, https://www.merriam-webster.com.

Example: Zack, a banker, leads workshops on financial literacy and budgeting for fellow Christians facing financial challenges. These workshops integrate biblical principles of stewardship, offering practical money management advice within the context of Christian beliefs.

11

The Judgment of Solomon

Solomon intermarried with Pharaoh the king of Egypt, and he took the daughter of Pharaoh and brought her to the city of David until he finished building his house, the house of Yahweh, and the walls of Jerusalem all around.

First Kings 3:1

THE ESTABLISHMENT of a marriage alliance between Solomon and the royal family of Egypt highlights the elevated status that the kingdom of Israel had achieved. This event suggests that the succession of the throne from King David to Solomon took place at a critical juncture in terms of international politics.

But the people *were* sacrificing on the high places, for the house for the name of Yahweh had not *yet* been built in those days. Solomon loved Yahweh, by walking in the statutes of David his father; only he *was* sacrificing and offering incense on the high places. So the king went to Gibeon to sacrifice, for the great high place *was* there. Solomon used to offer a thousand burnt offerings on that altar. Yahweh appeared to Solomon at Gibeon in a dream at night, and God said, "Ask what I should give to you." (3:2–5)

King Solomon ascended to the throne of Israel with a heart humbly inclined toward God, yearning for divine guidance above all else. He journeyed to the altar at Gideon and offered a thousand sacrifices to Yahweh. These offerings were a testament to his profound reverence for Him. The night following the sacrifice at Gideon, a divine encounter unfolded in his dream. God graciously offered to grant him any request he desired.

> Then Solomon said, "You have shown great loyal love with your servant David my father, as he walked before you in faithfulness and in righteousness and in uprightness of heart with you. You have shown him this great loyal love, and you have given a son to him who is sitting on his throne as *it is* this day. So then, O Yahweh, you are my God. You have made your servant king in place of David my father *though* I *am* a young boy. I do not know going out or coming in. Your servant *is* in the middle of your people whom you have chosen; a great people who cannot be counted or numbered because of abundance. Give to your servant a listening heart to judge your people, to discern between good and bad, because who is able to judge this, your difficult people?"
>
> The word was good in the eyes of *the* Lord that Solomon had asked this thing. And God said to him, "Because you have asked this thing and you did not ask for yourself *a long life* and you did not ask riches for yourself and you did not ask for the life of your enemies, but you have asked for yourself *the ability to make wise judgments*; behold, I do hereby do according to your word. I hereby give you a wise and discerning heart; there was no one like you before you, nor afterwards will one like you arise. Too, what you have not asked I give to you: both riches and honor, *so that* no man among the kings will be like you all of your days. If you will walk in my ways by keeping my statutes and my commandments, as David your father walked, then I will lengthen your days." (1 Kings 3:6–14)

Solomon asked for a listening heart to discern good and evil and to render fair justice. It wasn't earthly riches or power that he sought but a heart enriched with divine wisdom to govern his people righteously. In First Kings 3:9, the term "listening" is derived from the Hebrew word *shama*, denoting the capacity to hear, listen, and obey.[1] The word "heart" in the same verse is translated from the Hebrew word *leb*, signifying the inner person, moral character, or personal emotions.[2] In response to Solomon's humble request, God not only granted him the listening heart he asked for but also bestowed upon him divine wisdom and discernment that surpassed all others on the earth. The word "wise" in 3:12 originates from the Hebrew term *chakam*, an adjective representing practical wisdom and skills for various aspects of life, including technical work, administration, and learning.[3] The term "discerning" is rooted in the Hebrew word *binah*, an adjective form of *biyn*, denoting the capacity to exercise discernment in order to acquire understanding.[4] Even when Solomon himself wasn't aware of all his needs, God fully equipped him with all the necessary skills to rule the kingdom of Israel effectively. Furthermore, He granted him abundant wealth, honor, and even the promise of a long life.

> Then Solomon awoke, and look, *it was* a dream, and he came *to* Jerusalem and stood before the ark of the covenant of *the* Lord, and he offered burnt offerings and presented fellowship offerings, and he held a feast for all of his servants. (3:15)

Solomon presented burnt and fellowship offerings to Yahweh to show his reverence and gratitude for the divine grace he had received. He then hosted a joyful and abundant feast and invited all his servants to share in the celebration.

---

1 Warren W. Wiersbe, *The Wiersbe Bible Commentary: Old Testament* (Colorado Springs: David C. Cook, 2007), 620–622.

2 Bruce E. Winston, *Biblical Principles of Being an Employee in Contemporary Organizations* (Cham, Switzerland: Palgrave Macmillan, 2019), 31–34.

3 Winston, 31–34.

4 Wiersbe, 620–622.

> Then two prostitutes came to the king, and they stood before him. The one woman said, "Please my lord, I and this woman are living in one house, and I gave birth, with her in the house. It happened on the third day *after* my giving birth, this woman also gave birth, and we *were* together. There was not anyone with us in the house, only the two of us *were* in the house. Then the son of this woman died *in the* night because she laid on him. So she got up in the middle of the night, and she took my son from beside me while your servant was asleep, and she put him in her lap, and she put her dead son in my lap. When I got up in the morning to nurse my son, behold, he was dead! When I looked closely at him in the morning, behold, it was not my son whom I had borne." Then the other woman said, "No, for my son *is* the living one, and your son *is* the dead one." The other kept on saying, "No, for your son *is* the dead one, and my son *is* the living one," and so they argued in front of the king. Then the king said, "This one *is* saying, 'This *is* my son, the living one, but your son *is* the dead one,' and the other one keeps saying, 'But no! Your son *is* the dead one, and my son *is* living!'" (1 Kings 3:16–23)

Two women approached King Solomon, seeking his judgment on the custody of a baby boy. They resided in the same house and had given birth to baby boys just three days apart. Tragically, one of the women accidentally smothered her own son and attempted to hide her loss by switching her dead son with the other woman's baby. When the other woman woke up, she was horrified to find a lifeless infant who was not her own. The accused woman vehemently denied the charge and their dispute escalated before Solomon. With no evidence or witnesses, this was a case of one woman's word against the other's.

> So the king said, "Bring me a sword," and they brought the sword before the king. Then the king said, "Divide the living child into two, and give half to the one and half to the other." Then the woman whose son *was* the living one spoke to the king because her compassion was aroused for her son, and she

said, "Please, my lord, give her the living child, but certainly do not kill him!" The other one *was* saying, "As for me, so for you! Divide *him*!" Then the king answered and said, "Give the living child to her, and do not kill him; she *is* his mother." When all of Israel heard the judgment that the king had rendered, they *stood in awe* of the king, because they realized that the wisdom of God was in him to execute justice. (1 Kings 3:24–28)

As the tension mounted, Solomon commanded his attendant to fetch a sword. With the blade in hand, he strode purposefully toward the baby, fixing his gaze upon him. He then proposed to divide the baby in two, with each woman receiving an equal portion. One of the women immediately cried out in distress, begging him to spare the child's life, even if it meant surrendering him to the other woman. The other woman remained silent, showing no concern for the child's fate. Through the self-sacrificing love and treasuring of the child's life, the first woman revealed herself as the true mother. This story suggests that the source of King Solomon's legendary wisdom lay in his understanding of the profound love of the Creator.

What distinguishes Christianity from all other religions is the unconditional and self-sacrificing love of God for humanity. Throughout history, no other religion portrays a God who willingly sacrifices His own life to save humanity. This confirms His identity as the true God, for He treasures the life of those He created with His own breath and hands. He cherishes them with an intensity that defies earthly description.

The Creator's love for His creations can be likened to the love of a mother for her child, albeit on an infinitely grander scale. Just as a mother nurtures, protects, and unconditionally loves her child, the Creator tenderly watches over and cares for His creations. In both cases, there is an unbreakable bond, a connection that transcends words. The woman who showed indifference to the child's life symbolizes idolatrous gods that lead humanity toward destruction. Idolatrous gods do not cherish humanity because they did not bring them into existence. Instead, they derive perverse satisfaction from human sacrifice, sexual immorality, physical torture, financial extortion, and various other means of inflicting suffering upon their worshippers.

King Solomon resolved even the most complex disputes and rendered fair and wise judgments. People from all corners of the world, including monarchs, dignitaries, and scholars, journeyed to Jerusalem to witness the profound wisdom of King Solomon. Under his rule, Israel thrived, ushering in an unprecedented era of peace, prosperity, and glory that echoed through the ages. Israel, a nation traditionally rooted in agriculture, underwent a remarkable transformation into a thriving commercial hub (1 Kings 10:22). Numerous merchants flocked to the city of Jerusalem from far-flung places, crossing vast deserts and oceans to take part in its flourishing markets.

> King Solomon was greater than all the kings of the earth with respect to wealth and wisdom. All of the earth *was* seeking the presence of Solomon, to hear his wisdom which God had put in his heart. (10:23–24)

In the Book of Proverbs, King Solomon emphasized that wisdom comes from the fear of God. He reiterated this foundational truth three times within the book. He then explained that the fear of God guides individuals toward wisdom by setting them apart from evil, self-glorification, pride, and deception of the world.

> Fear of Yahweh *is* the beginning of knowledge;
> wisdom and instruction, fools despise.
> (Prov. 1:7)

> The start of wisdom is fear of Yahweh,
> and knowledge of the Holy One, insight.
> (Prov. 9:10)

> Fear of Yahweh *is* the instruction of the wise,
> and before honor *comes* humility.
> (Prov. 15:33)

> The fear of Yahweh *is* hatred of evil,
> pride, arrogance and an evil way.
> And I hate a mouth of perversity.
> (Prov. 8:13)

Along with the fear and reverence of God, the apostle James also encourages the believers to ask for wisdom from Him.

> Now if any of you lacks wisdom, let him ask for *it* from God, who gives to all without reservation and not reproaching, and it will be given to him. (James 1:5)

Second Timothy 3:16 reveals that by studying God's word, individuals gain discernment to distinguish right from wrong and act accordingly.

> All scripture *is* inspired by God and profitable for teaching, for reproof, for correction, for training in righteousness. (3:16)

The ABC (Abstract to Brick Concrete)

Wisdom—General Definition:[5]

- Ability to discern inner quantities and relationships, good sense, generally accepted belief.

Wisdom—Biblical Definition:

- Fear of God leading to the knowledge and skills needed to make the right choices for a successful, God-honoring life.

---

5 "Wisdom," Merriam-Webster.com, accessed October 23, 2023, https://www.merriam-webster.com.

Discernment—General Definition:[6]
- The quality of being able to grasp and comprehend what is obscure, an act of perceiving something.

Discernment—Biblical Definition
- Having the capacity to distinguish between right and wrong, wise and foolish; to acquire an understanding of difficult or complex issues.

The FAST (Focused, Actionable Steps to Take)

1. Identify the specific areas in which you need wisdom. Pray to God, seeking wisdom for these particular areas. Have faith that He will abundantly fulfill your needs.

   Example: Brianna identified a need for wisdom in her marriage as they faced disagreements on various fronts. She prayed in faith for wisdom to navigate these challenges in her relationship with her husband.

2. Study Scripture to acquire the knowledge and discernment to distinguish right from wrong and apply it in your actions.

   Example: After studying Exodus 20:12, which teaches the importance of honoring one's parents, Sam repented of his past disrespect toward his parents. He apologized and successfully reconciled with them. His action was guided by the knowledge and discernment he gained through studying the Scriptures.

---

6 "Discernment," Merriam-Webster.com, accessed October 23, 2023, https://www.merriam-webster.com.

12

The First Judge of Israel—Othniel

Joshua summoned all Israel, their elders, heads, judges, and officials, and he said to them, "I am old and well-advanced in years. . . . *Look! I have allotted to you these remaining nations as an inheritance for your tribes, from Jordan,* with *all the nations that I have cut off, to the Great Sea* in the west. *And Yahweh your God will push them* back before you *and drive them* out of your sight, *and you will possess their land, just as Yahweh your God promised to you."*

Joshua 23:2, 4–5

UPON ENTERING Canaan, the Israelites began driving out its inhabitants to claim the land. Over three decades, Joshua led the Israelites in conquering thirty-one Canaanite nations, stretching from the Jordan River to the Great Sea in the west (12:9–24). Before his death, Joshua urged the Israelite leaders to ensure the complete conquest of Canaan.

After the death of Joshua, the *Israelites* inquired of Yahweh, saying, "Who will go up first for us against the Canaanites to fight against them?" And Yahweh said, "Judah will go up. I hereby give the land into his hand." And Judah said to Simeon his brother, "Go up with me into my allotment, and let us fight against the Canaanites; then I too will go with you into your allotment." And Simeon went with him. And Judah went up, and Yahweh gave the Canaanites and the Perizzites into their hand, and they defeated ten thousand men at Bezek. At Bezek they came upon Adoni-bezek, and they fought against him and defeated the Canaanites and the Perizzites. And Adoni-bezek fled, but they pursued after him; they caught him and cut off *his thumbs and big toes*. Adoni-bezek said, "Seventy kings with *their thumbs and big toes* cut off used to pick up *scraps* under my table; just as I have done, so God has repaid to me. They brought him *to* Jerusalem, and he died there.

The descendants of Judah fought against Jerusalem, and they captured it, *put it to the sword*, and *set the city on fire*. Afterward the descendants of Judah pursued to fight against the Canaanites who were living in the hill country, the Negev, and the Shephelah. Judah went against the Canaanites living in Hebron (the former name of Hebron *was* Kiriath Arba). They defeated Sheshai, Ahiman, and Talmai. (Judg. 1:1–10)

The Canaanites took Joshua's passing as an opportunity to strike back, assuming that the leadership of Israel might falter in his absence. In response, Israel needed to demonstrate their unwavering strength through a resounding victory. The leaders of Israel convened in the town of Shiloh, seeking divine guidance through the high priest Phinehas. Yahweh commanded the tribe of Judah to charge into battle against the Canaanites with His assurance that He would deliver the land into their hands. The tribe of Judah fearlessly advanced, conquering the Canaanites and Perizzites and capturing the cities of Jerusalem, Negev, Shephelah, and Hebron. Their victorious march continued as they seized the city of Debir.

> And from there they went to the inhabitants of Debir (the former name of Debir *was* Kiriath Sepher). And Caleb said, "Whoever attacks Kiriath Sepher and captures it, I will give to him Acsah my daughter as a wife." Othniel son of Kenaz, the younger brother of Caleb, captured it, and he gave to him Acsah his daughter as a wife. When she came *to him*, she urged him to ask her father for a field. As she dismounted from the donkey, Caleb said to her, "*What do you want?*" And she said to him, "Give me *a gift*; you have given me the land of the Negev, and give me also a spring of water." And Caleb gave to her the upper and lower spring. (Judg. 1:11–15)

Caleb and his family hailed from the Kenizzite clan, believed to be descendants of Esau, Jacob's twin brother and a renowned hunter in his time (Josh. 14:14; Gen. 36:10–11). It's thought that Caleb's family may have integrated with the tribe of Judah during their stay in Egypt (Num. 13:6). It is important to note that the Kenizzites should not be confused with the Kenites, who have a different origin. The Kenites were related to Moses through his brother-in-law Hobab and played a role in guiding the Israelites in the wilderness (Gen. 15:19; Judg. 1:16). While the Kenizzites were renowned as skilled hunters, the Kenites were a nomadic group of metalworkers who introduced the craft of blacksmithing to the land of Canaan.[1]

Caleb promised his daughter Acsah's hand in marriage to anyone who could conquer the city of Kiriath-Sepher. Othniel, his nephew, achieved this feat and married Acsah. According to Jewish oral traditions, Othniel was a man consumed by the art of combat and the wisdom of the Scriptures. However, he showed little interest in accumulating wealth or material possessions. The pursuit of riches or worldly comforts seemed to have little appeal to him, as he was content with his humble way of life. However,

---

1 Warren W. Wiersbe, *The Wiersbe Bible Commentary: Old Testament* (Colorado Springs: David C Cook, 2007), 428–435.

his impoverishment greatly concerned Acsah.[2] Before leaving her father's house, she boldly approached him, requesting financial support. Caleb, understanding their dire financial situation, exceedingly fulfilled her request. Caleb and Othniel, despite being of Gentile origins, wholeheartedly worshipped and served Yahweh with unwavering devotion.

> For if indeed you turn back and join these remaining nations *among you*, and you intermarry with them, *marrying their women and they yours*, know for certain that Yahweh your God *will not continue to drive out* these nations from before you; they will be for you a snare and a trap, a whip on your sides and thorns in your eyes, until you perish from this good land that Yahweh your God has given to you. (Josh. 23:12–13)

With his last breath, Joshua imparted a final command to his people not to intermarry with the Canaanites. He warned them of the consequences that would come if they did not obey this command; God would cease to aid them in the battle to remove the remaining Canaanites from the land, leaving them as a constant source of affliction for the Israelites.

> The *Israelites* lived in the midst of the Canaanites, the Hittites, the Amorites, the Perizzites, the Hivites, and the Jebusites. They took their daughters as wives for themselves, and they gave their daughters to their sons, and they served their gods.
>
> The *Israelites* did evil in the eyes of Yahweh. They forgot Yahweh their God, and they served the Baals and the Asherah. And *the anger of Yahweh was kindled* against Israel, and he sold them into the hand of Cushan-Rishathaim, the king of Aram Naharaim; and the *Israelites* served Cushan-Rishathaim eight years. (Judg. 3:5–8)

Despite the forewarning, the Israelites intermarried with the Canaanites and adopted their deities. They abandoned their

---

2 Arthur Charles Hervey, *Judges* (London, UK: C. Kegan Paul and Company, 1881), 10–14.

God, Yahweh, in favor of worshipping pagan idols, the Baals and the Asherahs. As foretold, the remaining Canaanites became a severe affliction to them. The Arameans subjected the Israelites to harsh labor and mistreatment, and this oppression persisted for a grueling eight years. Cushan-Rishathaim was not the true name of the Aramean king but an Israelite satire meaning "double-wickedness" to underscore his harsh oppression of the Israelites. This satirical expression employed end rhymes to ridicule him.[3]

> The *Israelites* cried out to Yahweh, and Yahweh raised up a deliverer for the *Israelites* who delivered them, Othniel, son of Kenaz, Caleb's younger brother. The spirit of Yahweh came upon him and he judged Israel. He went out to war, and Yahweh gave Cushan-Rishathaim king of Aram into his hand, and *he prevailed over* Cushan-Rishathaim. So the land rested forty years. Then Othniel, son of Kenaz died. (Judg. 3:9–11)

Amid their brutal enslavement, the Israelites turned back to their God, Yahweh. Day and night, they cried out to Him for deliverance.

In response to their anguished plea, He called forth Othniel, the humble warrior, to rise to their rescue. Empowered by His Spirit, Othniel bravely led the charge into the battle against the Arameans. Through divine might and providence, he triumphed over the Aramean king Cushan-Rishathaim and his formidable army.

At the time of his divine calling as the first Judge of Israel, Othniel was elderly, possibly as old as 98.[4] Among many young Jewish men, the spirit of Yahweh came upon this elderly Gentile, Othniel. God did not count him out because of his advanced age and Gentile status. God doesn't call the qualified; he qualifies the called. Following the victory over the Arameans, Othniel

---
3 Robert H. O'Connell, *The Rhetoric of the Book of Judges* (Leiden, The Netherlands: E.J. Brill, 2014), 82–84.

4 Hervey, 30–31.

ruled Israel with enduring peace, a reign that lasted forty years until his passing.

The Hebrew term *shaphat*, translated as "judge" in Judges 3:10, carries a threefold meaning: First, it signifies the restoration of peace within a disrupted community, particularly for those who have suffered. Second, it embodies the enactment of judgment on those responsible for the disruption. And third, it can represent judgment as a means to exclude or even destroy those causing the disruption.[5] As the first Judge, Othniel served the Israelites by restoring harmony, enacting judgment, and, when necessary, taking decisive action against disruptors. His qualities of humility and modesty made him a respected and trusted figure among the Israelites. He humbly relied on Yahweh's guidance in leading the nation of Israel. His capacity to set aside personal ambition and ego enabled him to selflessly serve God and His people.

The Merriam-Webster English Dictionary defines "judge" as forming an opinion through careful consideration (see below). In contrast to its general definition, the word "judge" in the Bible is action-oriented and rooted in divine principles.

The ABC (Abstract to Brick Concrete)

Judge—General Definition:[6]

- To form an opinion about through careful weighing of evidence and testing of premises, to form an estimate or evaluation of, to hold as an opinion.

Judge— Biblical Definition:

- To restore peace within a disrupted community, particularly for those who have suffered, to enact judgment on

---

5   G. Johannes Botterweck and Helmer Ringgren, *Theological Dictionary of the Old Testament*, Vol. III (Grand Rapids: Eerdmans, 1974), 188–189.

6   "Judge," Merriam-Webster.com, accessed October 23, 2023, https://www.merriam-webster.com.

those responsible for the disruption, and to rule as a means to exclude or even destroy those causing the disruption.

The FAST (Focused, Actionable Steps to Take)

1. Engage with individuals who have been excluded from church fellowship and encourage others to include them in their activities.

   Example: Madison noticed that a church member with disabilities was being bullied in their Sunday school class. She approached the church member, forming a friendship and sitting with her during Sunday school sessions. She also talked to the other church members, explaining the importance of loving one another in Christ, and encouraged them to befriend her. Through her efforts, the bullying gradually ceased as the other church members embraced the message of the love of Christ, making Sunday school a more welcoming and supportive environment for all.

2. Support and provide resources for victims of injustice, such as socioeconomic disparities in health, education, and employment.

   Example 1: Emily volunteers in her local church once a week on Saturday afternoons, providing tutoring to students who have fallen behind in their studies and come from disadvantaged socioeconomic backgrounds.

   Example 2: Jim sets aside twenty minutes of his time every Tuesday evening to pray for Christians under severe persecution in countries practicing religious injustice.

13

The Unlikeliest Rescuer
—Jonah's Mission to the Enemy

> *In the fifteenth year of Amaziah the son of Jehoash king of Judah, Jeroboam the son of Jehoash king of Israel began to reign in Samaria,* **reigning** *forty-one years. But he did evil in the eyes of Yahweh; he did not depart from all the sins of Jeroboam the son of Nebat which he caused Israel to sin. He restored the boundary of Israel from Lebo-Hamath up to the sea of the Arabah, according to the word of Yahweh which he spoke by the hand of his servant Jonah the son of Amittai the prophet, who was from Gath-Hepher.*
>
> Second Kings 14:23–25

JONAH WAS A patriotic Israelite prophet who served the kingdom of Israel during the reign of King Joash and Jeroboam II. He was born in the town of Gath-Hepher, located a few miles north of Nazareth, belonging to the tribe of Zebulun.[1] According

---

1 James Hastings, John A. Selbie, and John C. Lambert, *A Dictionary of Christ and the Gospels*, Vol. II, Pt. 2 (Edinburgh, Scotland: T. & T. Clark, 1913), 847.

to Jewish tradition, Jonah is believed to be the son of the widow of Zarephath, who was miraculously resurrected by the prophet Elijah. However, it is important to note that Elijah's ministry preceded Jonah's by approximately 100 years, as he served during the reigns of Kings Ahab and Ahaziah. This significant time gap makes the traditional account of Jonah's lineage as the widow's son improbable.[2]

> The word of Yahweh came to Jonah the son of Amittai, saying, "Get up! Go to the great city Nineveh and cry out against her, because their evil has come up *before me*." But Jonah set out to flee toward Tarshish from *the presence of* Yahweh. He went down *to* Joppa and found a merchant ship going *to* Tarshish, and paid her fare, and went on board her to go with them toward Tarshish from *the presence of* Yahweh. (Jon. 1:1–3)

Yahweh commanded the patriot Jonah to forewarn the sinful city of Nineveh about the impending divine judgment. Notably, Nineveh was the capital of the Assyrian Empire, the foremost threat to the safety, independence, and prosperity of the kingdom of Israel.[3] Jonah held a fierce hostility toward the city of Nineveh, deeply rooted in his love and loyalty to his homeland. This frame of mind was far from an overreaction, as Assyria obliterated the nation of Israel in just four decades after this commandment and calling. One can easily grasp his fear that his action might contribute to the destruction of his own cherished family, city, and nation.

Rampant cruelty and wickedness characterized Nineveh, giving it a notorious title—"The City of Blood."[4] Nineveh was

---

2 Flavius Josephus, *The Genuine Works of Flavius Josephus, the Jewish Historian* (Boston: S. Walker, 1821), 344 (footnote).

3 Hal Seed, *Jonah: Responding to God in All the Right Ways* (n.c.: New Song Press, 2008), 109.

4 John F. Walvoord and Roy B. Zuck, eds., *Bible Knowledge Commentary: Old Testament* (Colorado Springs: David C. Cook, 1983), 1494.

considered "the center of savagery" even among the Assyrians.[5] Their wickedness had reached grotesque proportions, their cruelty had become unspeakable, and their moral degradation had sunk to unfathomable depths. It was a place where sexual immorality, idolatry, paganism, injustice, and violence thrived without remorse. Jonah felt a sense of righteous indignation, firmly convinced that the only just outcome for a society so far gone was destruction. In his eyes, it was the execution of divine justice, a reckoning long overdue for the savages. His conscience, that moral compass within him, echoed these sentiments, rendering its judgment that they were unworthy of forgiveness and redemption.

Jonah grappled with a moral conviction that saw the people of Nineveh as beyond redemption, a deep-rooted animosity born from years of enmity. He feared that their salvation might spell disaster for his own nation. This inner turmoil pushed him to defy God's command, and he set out on a journey far from his intended path. With a racing pulse, Jonah quickly boarded a ship bound for Tarshish, a destination in the exact opposite direction from Nineveh. In those days, it was customary to settle the fare upon reaching the destination port, but he paid his fare even before boarding the ship.[6] This unusual act of paying the fare in advance shows the urgency and desperation he felt to make a quick getaway. He was determined to go to great lengths to avoid this divine calling.

> Yahweh hurled a great wind upon the sea, and it was a great storm on the sea, and the merchant ship *was in danger of breaking up*. The mariners were afraid, and each cried out to his god. They threw the *contents* that were in the merchant ship into the

---

5 Miguel A. De La Torre, *Liberating Jonah: Forming an Ethics of Reconciliation* (Ossining, NY: Orbis Books, 2007), 11.

6 Matthew Poole, *Annotations Upon the Holy Bible*, Vol. 2 (London: Thomas Parkhurst, et al., 1700), 291.

sea to lighten it for them. And *meanwhile* Jonah went down into the hold of the vessel and lay down and fell asleep. The captain of the ship approached him and said to him, "Why are you *sound asleep*? Get up! Call on your god! Perhaps *your* god will take notice of us and we won't perish!" They said *to one another*, "Come, let us cast lots so that we may know on whose account this disaster *has come* on us!" They cast lots, and the lot fell on Jonah. So they said to him, "Please tell us whoever *is responsible that* this disaster *has come* upon us! What *is* your occupation? And from where do you come? What *is* your country? And from which people *are* you?" And he said to them, "I *am* a Hebrew, and I fear Yahweh, the God of heaven, who made the sea and the dry land." Then the men *were greatly afraid*, and they said to him, "What *is* this you have done?" because they knew that he *was* fleeing *from the presence of* Yahweh (because he had told them). So they said to him, "What shall we do to you so that the sea may quiet down for us?" because the sea *was growing more and more tempestuous*. (Jon. 1:4–11)

The ship Jonah had boarded sailed away from the shore, venturing into the vast Mediterranean Sea. As the ship ventured deeper into the open sea, a violent storm unleashed by God battered the vessel. Panic gripped all on board except Jonah, who knew the reason and the divine hand behind this tempest. The crew cast lots, which fell on Jonah, revealing him as the one responsible for the disaster that had befallen them. This revelation compelled the crew to confront Jonah, demanding an explanation and seeking guidance on how to quell the storm. The ferocious storm raged on, its waves assaulting the vessel as if they intended to shatter it.

Jonah confessed that he was fleeing from Yahweh, who had given him the mission to call upon the people of Nineveh to repent.

His love for his homeland, moral conviction, and animosity toward Nineveh made him feel it was impossible for him to continue serving Yahweh. The crew, perhaps expecting Jonah to fervently seek God's forgiveness or commit to fulfilling the divine task, were taken aback by his unexpected response.

> He said to them, "Pick me up and hurl me into the sea so that the sea may quiet down for you, because I know that on account of me this great storm *has come* upon you all." But the men rowed *hard* to bring the *ship* back to dry land, and they could not *do so* because the sea *was growing more and more tempestuous* against them. So they cried out to Yahweh, and they said, "O Yahweh! Please do not let us perish because of this man's life, and *do not make us guilty of innocent blood*, because you, O Yahweh, did what you wanted." And they picked Jonah up and hurled him into the sea, and the sea ceased from its raging. So the men feared Yahweh *greatly*, and they offered a sacrifice to Yahweh and *made* vows.
>
> And Yahweh provided a large fish to swallow up Jonah, and Jonah was in the belly of the fish for three days and three nights. (Jon. 1:12–17)

In the heart of the roaring gale, Jonah directed the crew to cast him into the churning waters, a sacrificial offering to quell the furious storm. He once again had chosen to flee from God, this time to the point of death. The crew, initially in disbelief, allowed some time, hoping that Jonah would come to his senses and seek divine forgiveness through repentance. They may have even beseeched Yahweh to extend His mercy to Jonah. As the storm grew fiercer, the crew had no option but to cast Jonah into the sea. As Jonah plunged into the water, the storm abruptly ceased. Amid the tumultuous sea storm, a colossal fish sent by Yahweh had been lurking all along, and it swiftly devoured Jonah. For three days and three nights, Jonah found himself inside the belly of this creature.

> And Jonah prayed to Yahweh his God from the belly of the fish and said,
>
> > "I called *from my distress* to Yahweh,
> >   and he answered me;

from the belly of Sheol I cried for help—
>   you heard my voice.
> You threw me *into the* deep,
>   into the heart of *the* seas,
>   and *the* sea currents surrounded me;
> all your breakers and your surging waves
>   passed over me.
> And I said, 'I am banished
>   from your sight;
> how *will I continue to look*
>   *on your holy temple?*'
> *The* waters encompassed me up to *my* neck;
>   *the* deep surrounded me;
>   seaweed was wrapped around my head.
> I went down to the foundations of *the* mountains;
>   the Underworld—its bars *were* around me forever.
> But you brought up my life from *the* pit,
>   Yahweh my God.
> When my life was ebbing away from me,
>   I remembered Yahweh,
> and my prayer came to you,
>   *to your holy temple.*
> Those who worship vain idols
>   forsake their loyal love.
> But I, with a voice of thanksgiving,
>   will sacrifice to you;
> I will fulfill what I have vowed.
>   Deliverance *belongs* to Yahweh!"

And Yahweh spoke to the fish, and it vomited Jonah out on the dry land. (Jon. 2:1–10)

In his act of disobedience, Jonah had firmly chosen death over absolute submission to Yahweh. Nevertheless, as he descended into the sea's depths, a powerful desire for life welled up within him, compelling him to cry out fervently for His deliverance. At that very moment, a colossal fish swiftly engulfed Jonah, plucking him from the jaws of death. Despite Jonah's belief that his disobedience had cast him out of God's presence, he realized that God still listened to his prayers. Jonah recognized that he had placed his love for his homeland, his moral compass, and his emotions above his allegiance to God, effectively turning them into idols. In his prayer, he openly confessed his actions and sought repentance for prioritizing these idols over Him, followed by giving gratitude and making vows to Him. The term "loyal love" in Jonah 2:8 comes from the Hebrew term *hesed*, signifying the faithful love and kindness of God toward His people.[7] The giant fish, following the divine command, gently disgorged Jonah onto dry land. Standing on the sunlit shores, Jonah relished the sweet fruits and drank refreshing water. His voice rose in heartfelt praise, expressing deep gratitude for the mercy and grace that had spared his life.

> And the word of Yahweh came to Jonah a second *time*, saying, "Get up! Go to Nineveh, the great city, and proclaim to it the message that I *am* telling you." So Jonah got up and went to Nineveh according to the word of Yahweh. Now Nineveh was *an extraordinarily great city*—a journey of three days *across*. Jonah began to go into the city on a journey of one day, and he cried out and said, "Forty more days and Nineveh will be demolished!" And the people of Nineveh believed in God, and they proclaimed a fast and put on sackcloth—from the greatest of them *to the least important.*
>
> And the news reached the king of Nineveh, and he rose from his throne and removed his royal robe, put on sackcloth, and sat in the ashes. And he had a proclamation made, and said,
>
> "In Nineveh, by a decree of the king and his nobles:
>
> "No human being or animal, no herd or flock, shall taste anything! They must not eat, and they must not drink water! And *the* human beings and the animals must be covered *with*

---

7 James Limburg, *Jonah* (Louisville: Westminster/John Knox, 1993), 70.

sackcloth! And they must call forcefully to God, and each must turn from his evil way and from the violence that is in his hands. Who knows? God may relent and change his mind and turn *from his blazing anger so that* we will not perish."

And God saw their deeds—that they turned from their evil ways—and God changed his mind about the evil that he had said *he would* bring upon them, and he did not do *it*. (Jon. 3:1–10)

God did not give up on Jonah or the people of Nineveh, so He sent Jonah back on the task he had initially failed. He employed the trials of the sea storm and the colossal fish to strengthen Jonah's faith, preparing him for this ministry in the city of Nineveh. Jonah embarked on a direct journey to Nineveh to deliver a warning about the impending divine judgment and call for repentance. Nineveh, situated approximately 500 miles (805 km) to the northeast of Israel, required about a week of travel on foot.[8] As he set foot in the city, a hushed awe fell upon the people. They recognized him as the prophet who served the king of Israel. Prophets from Israel were notorious for their hostility toward Gentile nations, and Jonah was a testament to this tradition.

Jonah delivered a warning of impending divine judgment and a call for repentance to the people of Nineveh. What made his message truly resonate with the Ninevites was their understanding that Jonah, who had previously shown hostility toward them, would not have undertaken a week-long journey to save them of his own accord. Furthermore, neighboring nations were well aware of the mighty God of Israel, famous for delivering the Israelites from Egypt, parting the Red Sea, defeating the Egyptian army, and gifting them the land of Canaan. Thus, the people of Nineveh, from the most influential to the most humble, were stirred to the core by his message. They swiftly cast aside their evil deeds and violence, donned sackcloth, and fasted, holding onto

---

8 Marci Ogrosky, *God's Cranky Prophets: Jonah & Habakkuk* (Bloomington, IN: WestBow Press, 2014), 26–27.

the hope that God might reconsider and grant them forgiveness, mercy, and grace. In response to this great repentance, God chose not to unleash the foretold calamity upon Nineveh.

> And this *was greatly displeasing* to Jonah, and *he became furious*. And he prayed to Yahweh and said, "O Yahweh, *was* this not *what I said* while I was in my homeland? Therefore *I originally fled* to Tarshish, because I knew that you *are* a gracious and compassionate God, slow to anger *and having great steadfast love*, and one who relents concerning calamity. And so then, Yahweh, please take my life from me, because *for* me death *is* better than life!" And Yahweh said, "*Is it right for you to be angry?*" (Jon. 4:1–4)

In 4:1, the expression "displeasing" comes from the Hebrew word *raah*, which can also be translated as evil, wickedness, and immorality in English.[9] His moral compass grappled with the sparing of the people in Nineveh, which he perceived as an issue of injustice, fueling his anger. He directly confronted God, expressing remorse for having delivered the warning to Nineveh. In his distress, Jonah lamented God's grace, compassion, and mercy. He even went as far as requesting God to take his life, as he found death more appealing than witnessing the continued existence of the Ninevites.

Jonah's anger stemmed from his sense of justice, rooted in his moral compass, which conflicted with God's decision to show mercy to the people of Nineveh. This interaction between Jonah and God highlights the human tendency to project their own beliefs and values onto divine matters and question His actions from their limited perspective. God's rhetorical question, probing Jonah's anger at His mercy upon the people of Nineveh, struck him. He had recently experienced God's forgiveness and mercy

---

9 Kari Storstein Haug, Interpreting Proverbs 11:18–31, Psalm 73, and Ecclesiastes 9:1–12 in Light of, and as a Response to, Thai Buddhist Interpretations (Leiden, The Netherlands: Brill, 2012), 192–194.

in his own life, and this question made him confront his own hypocrisy. He realized he was resentful of His mercy extended to others despite having received it himself.

> Jonah went out from the city and sat *down* east of the city, and he made for himself a shelter there. And he sat under it in the shade, *waiting to see* what would happen with the city. Yahweh God appointed a plant, and he made it grow up over Jonah to be a shade over his head, to save him from his discomfort. And Jonah *was very glad* about the plant. So God appointed a worm *at daybreak* the next day, and it attacked the plant, and it withered. *And when the sun rose*, God appointed a scorching east wind, and the sun beat down on Jonah's head and he grew faint. *And he asked that he could die* and said, "My death *is* better than my life!" So God said to Jonah, "*Is it right for you to be angry* about the plant?" And he said, "*It is right for me to be angry enough to die!*"
>
> But Yahweh said, "You are troubled about the plant, for which you did not labor nor cause it to grow. *It grew up in a night and it perished in a night*! And should I not be concerned about Nineveh, the great city, *in which there are* more *than one hundred and twenty thousand* people who do not know right from left, plus many animals?" (Jon. 4:5–11)

Jonah chose not to join in the celebration of divine forgiveness among the Ninevites. Instead, he sat in a shelter on the outskirts of the city to ponder the fate of the city. He hoped that the Ninevites' repentance would be short-lived, akin to the fleeting goodness of Ephraim. Yahweh appointed a plant to offer Jonah shade, providing him with great relief. However, the next morning, God sent a worm that destroyed the plant He had provided. As the day progressed, a hot wind blew away the clouds, exposing Jonah to the scorching sun. Overcome by the heat, Jonah pleaded with God to take his life, believing that death would be preferable to enduring the relentless sunlight.

God once more posed a rhetorical question to Jonah, asking if it was right for him to be so angry about the plant. In a startling reply, Jonah expressed that his anger was so deep that he wished for death. God emphasized the irony that Jonah cared deeply for a plant that he did not create or nurture, which lived for only a day while getting enraged at God for showing His mercy to all life in Nineveh He created and sustained. He counseled Jonah in that the people of Nineveh sinned, but they did so out of ignorance, lacking the knowledge of God's law.

Jonah's journey also reflects a profound psychological transformation. He initially held an egoistic perspective, primarily focused on his homeland, his moral compass, and personal emotions. However, when he received a divine mission, his focus shifted toward embracing God's values and perspective, essentially prioritizing God's will over his own. This transition marked a shift from egoism to what we can call *sanctification*, symbolizing a deeper connection with God.

Amid this transition, he found himself in an overwhelming state of confusion, torn between his own personal values, perspectives, and feelings and those aligned with God's divine will.[10] His initial response was an attempt to distance himself from God, thinking it might resolve the irreconcilable conflict he felt. However, during his flight, he encountered a stark realization of His omnipresence. It became evident to Jonah that God, as the Creator of the entire universe, including the heavens and the earth, cannot be escaped by anyone (Ps. 139:7–8). His "loyal love" and reverence for God kept him from rebelling, yet he couldn't bring himself to deny his own essence. This fierce internal battle intensified, plunging him into an identity crisis and ultimately driving him toward self-destructive actions.[11] Jonah had the crew

---

10 Kalman J. Kaplan, "Jonah and Narcissus: Self-integration versus self-destruction in human development," *Studies in Formative Spirituality*, Vol. 8, No. 1 (Pittsburgh: Duquesne University Press, 1987), 33–54.

11 Updesh Kumar, ed., *Handbook of Suicidal Behaviour* (Singapore: Springer Nature Singapore, 2017), 52–54.

cast him overboard and later pleaded with God for death twice in his shelter outside the city. Recognizing Jonah's dire straits, God intervened by protecting Jonah in a safe environment—the stomach of the giant fish—to work through his identity, moral, and emotional struggles.[12] Yahweh, the Sovereign Ruler of the universe, explained Himself to Jonah, a mere mortal, out of His exceptional kindness and love. His guidance culminated in Jonah's wholehearted submission to God's will, values, and divine perspective, underpinned by unshakable faith in His goodness.

The ABC (Abstract to Brick Concrete)

Loyal Love—General Definition:[13]

- Loyal: Unswerving, faithful, and lawful.
- Love: Strong affection for another arising out of personal ties or admiration, attachment, devotion.

Loyal Love—Biblical Definition:

- God's faithful love and kindness to His people.

Idol—General Definition:[14]

- Object of worship, false god, likeness of something, fallacy.

Idol—Biblical Definition:

- Anything placed above one's allegiance to God.

---

12 Kalman J. Kaplan, "Suicide and Suicide Prevention: Greek versus Biblical Perspectives," *OMEGA—Journal of Death and Dying*, Vol. 24, Issue 3, May 1992, 227–239.

13 "Loyal," "Love," Merriam-Webster.com, accessed October 23, 2023, https://www.merriam-webster.com.

14 "Idol," Merriam-Webster.com, accessed October 23, 2023, https://www.merriam-webster.com.

The FAST (Focused, Actionable Steps to Take)

1. Every morning, take a moment to personally praise God for His enduring love and kindness toward you.

   Example: Upon waking up, Nick offered a heartfelt prayer of gratitude to God, thanking Him for His faithful love and kindness. Specifically, Nick expressed his thankfulness for the strength God provided during a challenging meeting at work, where he successfully found a solution to a complex problem.

2. Reflect on your life and priorities on the first Sunday of each month. Examine aspects like material possessions, personal desires, and relationships to ensure you are not putting anything above your relationship with God.

   Example: On the first Sunday of each month, Laura set aside some quiet time for self-reflection and prayer. During these moments, she carefully assessed her life and identified any areas where her priorities were shifting away from her commitment to God. This month, Laura realized that her pursuit of career advancement had started to overshadow her spiritual growth. She was working long hours, often on Sundays, and felt a growing disconnect from her faith community. Recognizing this imbalance, she decided to make changes. She began attending church regularly and joined a small group for spiritual support.

14

Faith in Practice, Part 1
Triumphing over Trials
—James the Just

James, a slave of God and of the Lord Jesus Christ, to the twelve tribes in the dispersion. Greetings! Consider it *all joy, my brothers, whenever you encounter various trials,* because you *know that the testing of your faith produces endurance. Let endurance have* its *perfect effect, so that you may be mature and complete, lacking in nothing.*

James 1:1–4

And when his *[Jesus'] family* heard this, *they went out to restrain him, for they were saying, "He has lost his mind!"*

Mark 3:21

JAMES, AS THE half-brother of Jesus, understandably struggled to believe in His divinity, as illustrated in Mark 3:21. However, following Jesus' resurrection, James came to accept Him as the Christ. This transformation is evident in James 1:1, where he describes himself as a servant of God and Christ, affirming

His divinity. His plain and pragmatic personality is evident in the concise opening of this letter.

Under the persecution of Herod Agrippa I, many Jewish believers were driven away from the city of Jerusalem to many nations.[1] James penned this letter to guide them to remain steadfast in their saving faith amid rising persecution. He advised them to approach trials with joy, as enduring them would foster their spiritual maturity.

> Now if any of you lacks wisdom, let him ask for *it* from God, who gives to all without reservation and not reproaching, and it will be given to him. But let him ask for *it* in faith, without any doubting, for the one who doubts is like the surf of the sea, driven by the wind and tossed about. For that person must not suppose that he will receive anything from the Lord; *he is* a double-minded man, unstable in all his ways. (James 1:5–8)
>
> In everything taking up the shield of faith, with which you are able to quench all the flaming arrows of the evil one. (Eph. 6:16)

James advises those in trials to seek guidance from God on how to grow triumphantly through these challenging experiences. They need not concern themselves with their worthiness, as God's provision stems from His boundless generosity rather than their perceived deserving. While the exact origin of the saying is uncertain, it beautifully encapsulates the concept of His generosity: "Yahweh is the God of the open hand, not the God of the clenched fist." James passionately encourages fellow Christians to ask God with unwavering faith in His ability and willingness to provide. He even states that those lacking such faith shouldn't expect to receive anything from Him. James further describes the restless, unstable, and vulnerable status of those caught between faith and unbelief. Doubters are like sea waves, constantly moved and tossed by the wind, all because they lack the shield of faith.

---

[1] John MacArthur, NASB MacArthur Study Bible, 2nd Edition (Nashville: Thomas Nelson, 2020), 1695.

> Now let the brother of humble circumstances boast in his high position, but the rich person in his humiliation, because he will pass away like a flower of the grass. For the sun rises with its burning heat and dries up the grass, and its flower falls off, and the beauty of its appearance is lost. So also the rich person in his pursuits will wither away. (James 1:9–11)

> Now in those days prophets came down from Jerusalem to Antioch. One of them *named* Agabus stood up *and* indicated by the Spirit *that* a great famine was about to come over the whole inhabited earth (which took place in the time of Claudius). So from the disciples, *according to their ability to give*, each one of them determined to send *financial aid* for support to the brothers who lived in Judea, which they also did, sending *the aid* to the elders by the hand of Barnabas and Saul. (Acts 11:27–30)

In the early days of the church, Christians frequently faced marginalization from both Jewish and Gentile communities, placing them in a disadvantaged socioeconomic state. When the prophesied famine, as foretold by Agabus, struck the Roman Empire, their situation deteriorated considerably, as they were already enduring severe poverty.[2] James praises them for their faith and endurance in Christ, even in the face of great afflictions. When he advises them to "boast in [their] high position," he is commanding them to take pride in their spiritual maturity rather than indulging in worldly boasting. He points out that the wealthy, godless oppressors of Christians would ultimately face humiliation. James reminds them that the earthly glory of the rich is transitory and superficial, while the glory awaiting Christians is eternal and magnificent.

> Blessed *is* the person who endures testing, because *when he* is approved he will receive the crown of life that he has promised to those who love him. No one who is being tempted

---

2 Douglas J. Moo, *James: An Introduction and Commentary* (: InterVarsity Press, 2015), 91–95.

should say, "I am being tempted by God," for God *cannot be tempted* by evil, and he himself tempts no one. But each one is tempted *when he* is dragged away and enticed by his own desires. 15 Then desire, *after it* has conceived, gives birth to sin, and sin, *when it* is brought to completion, gives birth to death. (James 1:12–15)

In his exhortation for Christians to remain firm amid trials, James emphasizes the promise of eternal life for those who overcome the challenges of this earthly journey. Furthermore, he notes that the adversities act as the proving ground, unveiling the authenticity and strength of one's faith. When James says God never tempts, he means that God doesn't put believers in situations intending to lead them into wrongdoing or disobedience of His commands. Some individuals resist temptation and follow the path guided by His love and compassion, while unfortunately, others allow their desires to lead them to give in to sin.

Do not be deceived, my dear brothers. Every good gift and every perfect gift is from above, coming down from the Father of lights, with whom there is no variation or shadow of change. *By his* will he gave birth to us through the message of truth, so that we should be a kind of first fruits of his creatures. (James 1:16–18)

But according to his promise, we are waiting for new heavens and a new earth in which righteousness resides. (2 Pet. 3:13)

In his days Judah will be saved,
and Israel will dwell *in safety*,
and this *is* his name *by* which he will be called:
"Yahweh *is* our righteousness."

(Jer. 23:6)

In James 1:17, the word "gift" is derived from the Greek word *dosis*, which means the act of giving. However, the Greek word *dorea*, also translated as "gift" in the same verse, distinguishes the actual gift or thing given from *dosis*.[3] His point is that the same Creator who made those marvelous lights, the sun, moon, and stars with His hands is also the source of every good act of giving and the perfect gift itself. He further conveys the idea that everything created, including the celestial bodies, is subject to constant changes according to the laws and cycles established by the Creator. However, the Creator Himself does not change because He exists beyond His creation.

God brought forth His people, giving them life as His children through Christ, whose very essence is the Word of God (John 1:1–4). Believers, often referred to as the first fruits, symbolize the promise of a bountiful harvest and the beginning of a new creation of humanity through Christ. Just as humanity succumbed to sin at the time of Adam, believers represent the first of His new creation, reborn in Christ. They usher in a bountiful harvest through their labor of faith, much like the first and finest fruits offered to God. As a whole, Christians are also the first part of the new creation, as God has promised to create a new heaven and earth to dwell with those who have been reborn through Christ.

> Understand *this*, my dear brothers: every person must be quick to hear, slow to speak, slow to anger, for human anger does not accomplish the righteousness of God. (James 1:19–20)

> A man of anger will stir strife,
> and the owner of anger, much transgression.
> (Prov. 29:22)

James instructs believers to cultivate the habits of being prompt to listen, deliberate in speech, and measured in their emotional responses. This guidance is rooted in the understanding that anger often gives an opening to Satan, allowing hasty and

---

3 W.E. Vine and F.F. Bruce, *W.E. Vine's New Testament Word Pictures, Hebrews to Revelation* (Nashville: Thomas Nelson, 1984, 1996), 128.

unwise decisions to pave the way for conflicts and sins to manifest in the heat of impulsivity.

> Therefore, putting aside all moral uncleanness and wicked excess, welcome with humility the implanted message which is able to save your souls. (James 1:21)

> But if indeed our gospel is veiled, it is veiled among those who are perishing, among whom the god of this age has blinded the minds of the unbelievers, so that they would not see the light of the gospel of the glory of Christ, who is the image of God. (2 Cor. 4:3–4)

In James 1:21, "the implanted message" refers to the gospel, and its full understanding is concealed from those who receive it but continue to live immersed in sins, wickedness, and evil actions. Therefore, James calls on these believers to forsake their sinful habits and immoral conduct so they may benefit from its saving power.

> But be doers of the message and not hearers only, deceiving yourselves, because if anyone is a hearer of the message and not a doer, this one is like someone staring at *his own face* in a mirror, for he looks at himself and goes away and immediately forgets what sort of *person* he was. (1:22–24)

James compares believers who hear the word of God but don't act on it to a man who looks in a mirror and forgets his reflection when he walks away. In the first century, mirrors were made of highly polished bronze, silver, or even gold. They were a luxury, a prized possession beyond reach for many. Nonetheless, their reflections were poor, with hazy definitions, demanding considerable effort and time for one to study their reflection in the mirror.[4] This man spent a lot of time and effort to find a smudge on his nose in the mirror, but it was all in vain because he didn't

---

4 J.D. Douglas, Merrill C. Tenney, and Moises Silva, *Zondervan Illustrated Bible Dictionary* (Grand Rapids: Zondervan, 1987, 2011), 959.

bother to clean it off. While his forgetfulness might seem absurd, a man who gazes into the mirror with no intention of taking action, regardless of what he sees, would indeed forget it immediately afterward. James employs this analogy to underscore that knowing Christ's teachings without putting them into practice in one's life would not lead to spiritual maturity.

> But the one who looks into the perfect law of liberty and continues *to do it*, not being a forgetful hearer but a doer who acts, this one will be blessed *in what he does*.
>
> If anyone thinks he is religious, *although he* does not bridle his tongue but deceives his heart, this person's religion *is* worthless. Pure and undefiled religion in the sight of our God and Father is this: to look after orphans and widows in their affliction, *and* to keep oneself unstained by the world. (James 1:25–27)

"The perfect law of liberty" is a principle that liberates Christians from seeking righteousness through their own efforts and allows them to exceed the requirements of the law through Christ's mercy. Within this law of liberty, believers are called to follow the teachings of Christ under the guidance of the Holy Spirit. Implementing His teachings in everyday life includes acts of charity and compassion toward fellow Christians in need, such as orphans and widows, as well as maintaining holiness by distancing oneself from worldly influences. The following Scriptures delve into this transformative process, known as sanctification.

> When the Lord has washed away the filth of the daughters
> > of Zion
> > and cleansed the blood of Jerusalem from her midst
> by a spirit of judgment
> > and by a spirit of burning.
>
> (Isa. 4:4)
>
> Some of you were these *things*, but you were washed, but you were sanctified, but you were justified in the name of the Lord Jesus and by the Spirit of our God. (1 Cor. 6:11)

Isaiah 4:4, authored by Isaiah, bears a striking resemblance to First Corinthians 6:11, penned by the apostle Paul, despite being separated by approximately 600 years. Isaiah composed his verse before the commencement of Christ and the Holy Spirit's influence on humanity, while Paul's writing came after their ministry had begun.

Both Isaiah 4:4 and First Corinthians 6:11 outline a two-step process where believers must first undergo an instantaneous cleansing by the blood of Christ, followed by a gradual sanctification by the Holy Spirit. The Holy Spirit distinguishes those whose sins have been cleansed by Christ from non-believers. He exclusively indwells those whom Christ has purified, guiding them through the process of sanctification.

> I have given them your word, and the world has hated them, because they are not of the world just as I am not of the world. I do not ask that you take them out of the world, but that you protect them from the evil one. They are not of the world, just as I am not of the world. Sanctify them in the truth—your word is truth. Just as you sent me into the world, I also have sent them into the world. And for them I sanctify myself, so that *they* themselves also may be sanctified in the truth. (John 17:14–19)

The Oxford English Dictionary defines sanctification as the process of making something holy or giving it official approval.[5] In the Gospel of John, Christ prayed fervently for the sanctification of His followers. He emphasized that He sanctifies Himself for their sake and underscored that He is not of this world, just as His disciples are not. His prayer was to set them apart from the world, creating a wall between His followers and the worldly influences of sin, impurity, and unholiness. This passage describes sanctification as a process of detachment from the world's sway.

---

5 Maurice Waite, *Pocket Oxford English Dictionary* (Oxford, UK: Oxford University Press, 2013), 807.

The ABC (Abstract to Brick Concrete)

Sanctification—General Definition:[6]

- The state of being set apart to a sacred purpose or to religious use.

Sanctification—Biblical Definition:

- The process guided by the Holy Spirit of detaching believers from the world's sway and transforming them into pure, spiritually mature, Christlike individuals.

The FAST (Focused, Actionable Steps to Take)

Regularly study the Scriptures to maintain your focus on God. His Word equips individuals with the knowledge, moral foundation, and spiritual strength necessary to resist worldly influences.

Example: Beryl studies a chapter of the Bible over two days and repeats this process throughout the year. On day one, she reads the chapter both in the morning and the afternoon. On day two, she takes some time to meditate and reflect on what she has read. She then jots down her reflections in her devotional diary.

---

6 "Sanctification," Merriam-Webster.com, accessed October 23, 2023, https://www.merriam-webster.com.

15

Faith in Practice, Part 2

Connecting Belief to Action
—James the Just

My brothers, do not hold your faith in our glorious Lord Jesus Christ with partiality. For if someone enters into your assembly in fine clothing with a gold ring on his finger, and a poor person in filthy clothing also enters, and you look favorably on the one wearing the fine clothing and you say, "Be seated here in a good place," and to the poor person you say, "You stand or be seated there by my footstool," have you not made distinctions among yourselves and become judges with evil thoughts? Listen, my dear brothers! Did not God choose the **poor of the world** *to be* **rich in faith, and heirs of the kingdom that he has promised to those who love him?** *But you have dishonored the poor! Are not the rich exploiting you and they themselves dragging you into the courts? Do they themselves not blaspheme the good name* **of the one to whom you belong?** *However, if you carry out the royal law according to the scripture, "You shall love your neighbor as yourself," you are doing well. But if you show partiality, you commit sin,* **and thus** *are convicted by the law as transgressors.*

James 2:1–9

> *To execute judgment against all, and to convict all the ungodly concerning all their ungodly deeds that they have committed in an ungodly way, and concerning all the harsh things that ungodly sinners have spoken against him. These* people *are grumblers, discontented, proceeding according to their desires, and their mouths speaking pompous* words, showing partiality to gain an advantage.
>
> Jude 15–16

> *Peter opened* his *mouth* and *said, "In truth I understand that God is not one who shows partiality."*
>
> Acts 10:34

> *For* there *is no partiality with God.*
>
> Romans 2:11

JAMES THE JUST teaches Christians not to discriminate against the poor because of their lack of wealth. He illustrates a pattern of discrimination where the rich receive preferential treatment while the poor are often left without even a proper seat. He emphasizes that the poor were also chosen by God as heirs of His kingdom. He also reminds the people that the poor are their neighbors, whom they should love as themselves. He strongly condemns such discrimination rooted in worldly standards such as wealth, social status, or nationality, deeming it as evil.

Similarly, Jude also identifies those who show partiality as ungodly sinners. This teaching is not new, as it aligns with the principles found in the Mosaic Law (Exod. 23:3; Deut. 1:17; 10:17; 16:19; Lev. 19:15). Teachings against discrimination also abound in the book of Proverbs (Prov. 18:5; 22:2; 24:23; 28:21). Paul and Peter also explicitly stated that in God, there is no partiality. This impartial nature of God is consistently emphasized throughout the Scriptures (2 Chron. 19:7; Gal. 2:6; Eph. 6:9; Col. 3:25).

> For whoever keeps the whole law but stumbles in one *point only* has become guilty of all *of it*. For the one who said "Do not commit adultery" also said "Do not murder." Now if you do not commit adultery but you do murder, you have become a transgressor of the law. Thus speak and thus act as those who are going to be judged by the law of liberty. For judgment *is* merciless to the one who has not practiced mercy. Mercy triumphs over judgment. (James 2:10–13)

> But the one who looks into the perfect law of liberty and continues *to do it*, not being a forgetful hearer but a doer who acts, this one will be blessed *in what he does*. (1:25)

James explains that under the Mosaic Laws, violation of a single law, regardless of adherence to the other 612, disqualifies an individual from achieving righteousness. It functions as an "all-or-nothing" system, making selective obedience to certain laws insufficient. He instructs Christians to embrace the law of liberty, which enables them not only to meet but to surpass its requirements through the mercy of Christ. It is named the law of liberty because it liberates them from the burden of seeking righteousness solely through their own human efforts. Within the framework of this new law, believers can authentically live out God's principles by placing their faith in Christ and relying on the work of the Holy Spirit (John 8:36; 13:34–35; Matt. 22:36–40). James also advises Christians to be merciful and nonjudgmental toward each other, emphasizing that they all operate under the law of liberty due to His mercy.

> What is the benefit, my brothers, if someone says *that he* has faith but does not have works? That faith *is* not able to save him, *is it*? If a brother or a sister is poorly clothed and lacking food for the day, and one of you should say to them, "Go in peace, keep warm and *eat well*," but does not give them what

is necessary for the body, what *is* the benefit? Thus also faith, if it does not have works, is dead by itself. (James 2:14–17)

James provides clarity that saving faith is not merely a profession but a way of living. He underscores that while believers are saved by faith alone, this saving faith is invariably accompanied by good works. His message emphasizes the pivotal role that works play in demonstrating the authenticity of their faith. James uses an example of someone coming across a loved one in need of clothing and food but offering empty words without taking real action. In this context, he is emphasizing that genuine love is missing. He then connects this example to followers of Christ who may express their love for Him but fail to follow His teachings, suggesting that their professed love may not necessarily lead to the saving faith they claim to have.

> But someone will say, "You have faith and I have works." Show me your faith apart from your works, and I will show you my faith by my works. You believe that God is one; you do well. Even the demons believe, and shudder! But do you want to know, O foolish person, that faith apart from works is useless? (2:18–20)

James rejects the idea that saving faith and works can be entirely separate. He points out that even demons believe in God, but their faith doesn't result in their salvation or eternal life. He contends that faith without corresponding works is ultimately pointless. Saving faith and deeds are inseparable, much like a spring and its source. Just as the source feeds the spring, giving it life, saving faith fuels our actions with compassion and kindness. Without this source, the spring would run dry, and likewise, without saving faith, our deeds would lack the life-giving essence of love and goodness. It's impossible to have saving faith and not witness the deeds it inevitably leads to, for they are intrinsically intertwined, like the source and the spring, inseparable and essential.

> Was not Abraham our father justified by works *when he* offered up his son Isaac on the altar? You see that faith was working together with his works, and by the works the faith was perfected. The scripture was fulfilled that says, "Abraham believed God, and it was credited to him for righteousness," and he was called God's friend. You see that a person is justified by works and not by faith alone. (James 2:21–24)

When Adam and Eve consumed the forbidden fruit from the Tree of Knowledge of Good and Evil, they instantly acquired their own moral compass, which they termed "conscience." However, this intuitive guide sometimes contradicted divine moral standards. Over time, as sin drove a wedge between God and humanity, people increasingly followed their conscience's judgments of right and wrong, departing from divine moral principles.

In contrast, Abraham's unshakable faith enabled him to defy the constraints of his own conscience and obediently trust in God's goodness. God tasked Abraham with something that, by human standards, would be deemed morally objectionable. Nevertheless, Abraham demonstrated that humanity could be restored to its original design through faith. His triumph over the limitations of conscience through faith served as a beacon of hope for humanity's reconciliation with God.

> Likewise was not Rahab the prostitute also justified by works *when she* welcomed the messengers and sent *them* out by a different route? For just as the body without the spirit is dead, so also faith without works is dead. (2:25–26)

In the first century, Abraham was held in high regard as the father of faith among the Jews. James, in his writings, positions Abraham alongside Rahab, a Canaanite prostitute, as an exemplar of faith for the followers of Christ. This juxtaposition was a daring move, as it challenged conventional beliefs and could have posed a threat to him from groups like the Pharisees and

Sadducees, who staunchly upheld established Jewish traditions. Nevertheless, James, a man who practiced what he preached, makes this bold pairing to demonstrate there is no partiality in Christ, regardless of worldly standards such as social status, nationality, or wealth. The love of Christ goes beyond earthly distinctions to unite all those He has chosen.

The ABC (Abstract to Brick Concrete)

Law of Liberty—General Definition:[1]

- Law: A binding custom or practice of a community; a rule of conduct or action prescribed or formally recognized as binding or enforced by a controlling authority; the whole body of such customs, practices, or rules.

- Liberty: The quality or state of being free; the power to do as one pleases; right or immunity enjoyed by prescription or by grant; permission to go freely within specified limits.

Law of Liberty—Biblical Definition:

- A principle that liberates Christians from seeking righteousness through their own efforts and allows them to surpass the law's requirements through Christ's mercy.

The FAST (Focused, Actionable Steps to Take)

As part of your daily Christian journey within the law of liberty, begin by engaging in fellowship with fellow believers, fostering an environment of forgiveness and understanding within your community.

---

1 "Law," "Liberty," Merriam-Webster.com, accessed October 23, 2023, https://www.merriam-webster.com.

Example 1: In the morning, Edward began his day by offering thanksgiving to God for His boundless mercy and forgiveness. Later in the day, when his coworker accidentally lost an important document, Edward chose to forgive, guided by the principles of the law of liberty and his deep appreciation for God's grace. He extended the same mercy he had received, understanding that forgiveness and understanding were vital components of living in accordance with the law of liberty.

Example 2: Every day, as Aubrey's day comes to an end, she takes a moment to reflect on her actions. She carefully evaluates how effectively she has incorporated forgiveness and mercy into her interactions. She's mindful of aligning her behavior with the guiding principles of the law of liberty. This daily reflection helps her continually practice forgiveness and mercy in her life, living in harmony with the teachings of this law.

16

Beware the Wolves

The elder, to the elect lady and her children, whom I love in truth—and not I alone, but also all those who know the truth—because of the truth that resides in us and will be with us **forever.** *Grace, mercy, peace will be with us from God the Father and from Jesus Christ the Son of the Father in truth and love.* **I was very glad** *because I found* **some** *of your children walking in* **the** *truth, just as* **the Father commanded us.**

Second John 1–4

JOHN THE APOSTLE addresses his letter to a faith-based family deeply cherished and respected by fellow Christians. Whether this family represents real individuals or serves as a metaphorical illustration for the church, what remains significant is that it symbolizes a community bound together by faith, love, and their shared devotion to Christ.

> Now I ask you, lady (not as *if I were* writing a new commandment to you, but *one* that we have had from the beginning), that we should love one another. This is love: that we walk according to his commandments. This is the commandment,

just as you have heard from the beginning, so that you should walk in it. (2 John 5–6)

John, known as the Apostle of Love, centered his teaching on the importance for Christians to love one another. In this letter, he encourages the family to keep nurturing and sharing this profound love they have in Christ.

> For many deceivers have gone out into the world, those who do not confess Jesus Christ coming in *the* flesh. This person is the deceiver and the antichrist! Watch yourselves so that you do not lose what we have worked for, but receive a full reward. Everyone who goes too far and does not remain in the teaching of Christ does not have God. The one who remains in the teaching—this person has both the Father and the Son. If anyone comes to you and does not bring this teaching, do not receive him into *your* house and do not speak a greeting to him, because the one who speaks a greeting to him shares in his evil deeds. (7–11)

As the gospel spread, false teachers emerged, denying the incarnation of Christ. John warns that this false teaching if embraced within the Christian community, could threaten the unity they worked hard to establish. He refers to the false teachers as "antichrists" to emphasize their role in leading Christians astray. According to the Heinemann English Dictionary, false teachers are individuals characterized as being untrue, inaccurate, deceptive, and unfaithful in their teaching.[1] In verse 9, the Greek word *proago*, translated as "too far," signifies "progressive," individuals whose teachings markedly deviate from canonical doctrines of Christianity.[2] John advises the family to

---

1 Martin Manser et al., eds., *Heinemann English Dictionary* (Oxford: Heinemann, 2001), 363.

2 Prosper Grech, *An Outline of New Testament Spirituality* (Grand Rapids: Eerdmans, 2011), 123.

exercise caution against such teachers so they would not be led astray from the true teaching of Christ. He implores the family to refrain from any interaction, not even a greeting, with the false teachers. This drastic measure was taken to protect the family from their deceptive influence.

Gnosticism was a religious practice that asserted salvation through the knowledge of the divine and the universe. Gnostics believed such knowledge could only be obtained through direct spiritual revelation. Gnostics also rejected the belief that Jesus was both fully God and fully human. It is possible that the warning in this letter was aimed at the preachers tainted with Gnosticism.[3]

> *Although* I have many *things* to write to you, I do not want *to do so* by means of paper and ink, but I hope to be with you and to speak *face to face*, so that your joy may be complete. The children of your elect sister greet you. (2 John 12–13)

As the letter draws to a close, the apostle John warmly expresses his heartfelt desire to visit the family in person. His wish is to share in the joyous communion of fellow believers in Christ, to strengthen their bonds, and to personally partake in the spiritual fellowship that unites them in their faith.

The ABC (Abstract to Brick Concrete)

False Teachers—General Definition:[4]

- *False:* intentionally untrue; adjusted or made so as to deceive; intended or tending to mislead.
- *Teacher:* one who instructs by precept, example, or experience.

---

3 Craig A. Evans, *The Bible Knowledge Background Commentary: John's Gospel, Hebrews–Revelation* (Colorado Springs: David C. Cook, 2005), 176.

4 "False," "Teacher," Merriam-Webster.com, accessed October 23, 2023, https://www.merriam-webster.com.

False Teachers—Biblical Definition:
- Individuals whose teachings markedly deviate from the biblical doctrines of Christianity.

The FAST (Focused, Actionable Steps to Take)

When you learn about God's word from someone else, be sure to carefully compare it with Scripture to ensure consistency.

Example: Jason attended a church in the new town he had recently moved to. He took notes on the key points from the preacher's sermon. After returning home, he compared his notes to the Bible and was pleased to find them consistent. As a result, Jason decided to return to the same church next week, confident that the pastor's teachings aligned with Scripture.

17

Blessed Beyond Measure—Abraham

Yahweh said to Abram, "Go out from your land and from your relatives, and from the house of your father, to the land that I will show you. And I will make you a great nation, and I will bless you, and I will make your name great. And you will be a blessing. And I will bless those who bless you, and those who curse you I will curse. All families of the earth will be blessed in you." . . . For I have chosen him [Abraham], that he will command his children and his household after him that they will keep the way of Yahweh, to do righteousness and justice, so that Yahweh may bring upon Abraham that which he said to him.

Genesis 12:1–3; 18:19

Understand that the ones who have faith, these are sons of Abraham. And the scripture, foreseeing that God would justify the Gentiles by faith, proclaimed the good news in advance to Abraham: "In you all the nations will be blessed." So then, the ones who have faith are blessed together with Abraham who believed. . . . If you are Christ's, then you are Abraham's offspring, heirs according to the promise.

Galatians 3:7–9, 29

APPROXIMATELY 4,000 years ago, Yahweh called upon a man named Abraham, endowing him with a divine blessing. This blessing designated him as the foundational source of blessings for all of humanity, with this divine grace extending through his descendants. Genesis 18 revealed that the fulfillment of the promised blessing hinges on Abraham and his descendants living their lives in righteousness and justice as divinely called.

This divine calling and the blessings it carries hold profound relevance for Christian believers. Just as Abraham received these blessings through unwavering faith, individuals of faith, akin to Abraham, become recipients of His abundant blessings and heirs to His promises. This draws attention to the call for Christians to live a life rooted in righteousness and justice.

The Heinemann English Dictionary defines "righteousness" as being morally right, truthful, just, and straightforward.[1] The Hebrew for "righteousness" is *tsedeq*, a word denoting what is deemed the normative, natural, or ideal state.[2] Yahweh created humankind in His image to bear His likeness and reflect His glory; hence, the natural course for humans is to manifest His divine qualities in their words and deeds (Gen. 1:27). This encompasses living with compassion, extending grace, showing meekness, practicing love, upholding faithfulness, and standing for justice (Exod. 34:6–7). Righteousness, in this sense, is a profound calling to mirror the divine, to align one's character with the very essence of God.

However, as human history unfolded, all fell short of this divine calling to be righteous, succumbing to sin (Ps. 53:3). These transgressions created a chasm between humanity and God, resulting in the loss of touch with the divine virtues (Isa. 59:2).

---

1   Martin Manser, et al., eds., Heinemann English Dictionary (Oxford: Heinemann, 2001), 869.

2   Darwin Chandler, *The Royal Law of Liberty: Living in Freedom Under Christ's Law of Love* (Bloomington, IN: Trafford Publishing, 2003), 22.

> For in this way God loved the world, so that he gave his one and only Son, in order that everyone who believes in him will not perish, but will have eternal life. . . . The one who believes in him is not judged, but the one who does not believe has already been judged, because he has not believed in the name of the one and only Son of God. (John 3:16, 18)

> Therefore, *because we* have been declared righteous by faith, we have peace with God through our Lord Jesus Christ. . . . God demonstrates his own love for us, *in* that *while* we were still sinners, Christ died for us. Therefore, by much more, *because we* have been declared righteous now by his blood, we will be saved through him from the wrath. (Rom. 5:1, 8–9)

As humanity was cast adrift, enslaved to the dominion of sin, committing deeds of darkness and evil, His boundless love for them shone through. God sent His only Son, Christ, to atone for the sins of humanity. Through faith in Christ, those who believed became justified and declared righteous in the sight of God. This liberation shattered the chains of sin, evil, and wickedness, freeing them from the depths of suffering and despair.

> Therefore, brothers, *since we* have confidence for the entrance into the sanctuary by the blood of Jesus, *by the* new and living way which he inaugurated for us through the curtain, that is, his flesh, and *since we have* a great priest over the house of God, let us approach with a true heart in the full assurance of faith, our hearts sprinkled *clean* from an evil conscience and our bodies washed with pure water. (Heb. 10:19–22)

> But you are not in the flesh but in the Spirit, if indeed the Spirit of God lives in you. But if anyone does not have the Spirit of Christ, this person *does not belong to him.* But if Christ *is* in you, the body *is* dead because of sin, but the Spirit *is* life because of righteousness. (Rom. 8:9–10)

By the blood of Christ, they were cleansed of sin and ushered into the very presence of God. This divine purification wrought a profound reconciliation, restoring their relationship with God. As they became the righteousness of God, the Holy Spirit came to dwell within them, serving as their advocate, interceding between them and God, and imparting strength to fulfill their divine calling to righteousness (John 14:16–17; Rom. 8:26–27).

> *As they* looked intently at him [Stephen], all those who were sitting in the Sanhedrin saw his face *was* like the face of an angel. (Acts 6:15)
>
> We all, with unveiled faces, reflecting the glory of the Lord, are being transformed into the same image from glory into glory, just as from the Lord, the Spirit (2 Cor. 3:18)

Through the new way through Christ, His followers were transformed back to the image of God as the apostle Paul testified in Second Corinthians 3:18. Stephen, a deacon martyred in Jerusalem, was described as having a countenance resembling that of an angel. This angelic visage likely symbolized his righteousness, reflecting divine attributes and the glory of God through his appearance. In the book of Galatians, the apostle Paul lists the characteristics of the fruit of the Spirit as follows: love, joy, peace, patience, kindness, goodness, faithfulness, gentleness, and self-control (Gal. 5:22–23). These qualities reflect the attributes of Yahweh that Christian believers, as the righteous ones, should strive to manifest in their lives.

> I am able to do nothing by myself. Just as I hear, I judge, and my judgment is just, because I do not seek my *own* will, but the will of the one who sent me. (John 5:30)
>
> Therefore you pray in this way:
> > Our Father who is in heaven,
> > may your name be treated as holy.
> > May your kingdom come,
> > may your will be done
> > > on earth as *it is* in heaven.

> Give us today our daily bread,
> and forgive us our debts,
>> as we also have forgiven our debtors.
> And do not bring us into temptation,
> but deliver us from the evil one.
> (Matt. 6:9–13)
>
> And going forward a little he fell down on his face, praying and saying, "My Father, if it is possible, let this cup pass from me. Nevertheless, not as I will, but as you *will*." (26:39)

The Hebrew term *mishpat* is translated as "justice" in the English Bible.³ *Mishpat* signifies a devoted pursuit of the divine will of God through wholehearted submission, transcending personal desires. Christ taught His disciples to pray for God's will to be done on earth as it is in heaven. As the moment of His crucifixion approached, Christ prayed for God's will to prevail over His own. Through this alignment with the divine will of God, Christians can partake in His wonderful work. Earthly justice, as noted in the Heinemann English Dictionary, is defined as being fair or impartial. The difference between the biblical definition of the word "justice" and its earthly counterpart is significant.⁴

> David reigned over all of Israel, and he was administering justice and righteousness for all his people. (2 Sam. 8:15)
>
> *He brought them before the king of Moab*, and they stayed with him all the days David was in the stronghold. Then Gad the prophet said to David, "You should not stay in the stronghold; leave and go into the land of Judah." So David left and came *to* the forest of Hereth. (1 Sam. 22:4–5)
>
> Mephibosheth the son of Jonathan, the son of Saul, came to David. He fell on his face and did obeisance. David said, "Me-

---

3 Chandler, 22.
4 Manser, 554.

phibosheth," and he said, "*I am ready to serve you.*" Then David said to him, "Don't be afraid, for *I will certainly show* loyal love to you for the sake of Jonathan your father, and I will restore to you all the lands of Saul your father. You shall always eat food at my table." (2 Sam. 9:6–7)

> You prepare before me a table
> in the presence of my oppressors.
> You anoint my head with oil;
> my cup *is* overflowing.
> (Ps. 23:5)

King David exemplifies a life deeply rooted in righteousness and justice. He mirrors divine attributes like kindness, compassion, and faithfulness. His generosity toward Mephibosheth, Jonathan's son, highlights these qualities. When David took refuge in Moab to escape King Saul's pursuit, God's prophet directed him to return to Judah. Without hesitation, David wholeheartedly submitted to God's divine will, entrusting his life entirely to the hands of the Almighty. Whether facing small everyday choices or major decisions that would shape the fate of Israel, he unwaveringly placed God's will above his own desires or beliefs. Much like King David, followers of Christ should strive to live in accordance with righteousness and justice, upholding the divine calling and spiritual legacy inherited from Abraham. This will release the stream of abundant blessings that will flow through their lives to the rest of the world. King David bore witness to these blessings that overflowed beyond measure in Psalm 23:5.

The ABC (Abstract to Brick Concrete)

Righteousness—General Definition:[5]

- Being morally right, truthful, just, and straightforward.

---

[5] Manser, 869.

Righteousness—Biblical Definition:

- Displaying the qualities of Yahweh in one's words and actions; this involves living with compassion, extending grace, showing meekness, practicing love, upholding faithfulness, and standing for justice.

Justice—General Definition:[6]

- Being fair or impartial.

Justice—Biblical Definition:

- A devoted pursuit for the divine will of God through wholehearted submission, transcending personal desires.

The FAST (Focused, Actionable Steps to Take)

1. Show love and compassion in your interactions with the people you encounter in your daily life.

   Example 1: Mary cooks dinner for her parents once a week as a way of showing her love for them.

   Example 2: Jessica gives her full attention when her classmates speak to her, showing that she values their thoughts and feelings.

2. Set aside your time and resources to serve those in need within your community.

   Example 1: Candice often drives an elderly woman who lives by herself to her medical appointments to ensure she gets the care she needs.

   Example 2: Kelly provides groceries once a week for a friend who was unexpectedly laid off and is going through financial hardship.

---

6 Manser, 554.

18

Invincible Hero of God—Asa

Abijah slept with his ancestors, and they buried him in the city of David. And Asa, his son, became king in his place. In his days the land was at rest for ten years. Asa did that which was good and right in the eyes of Yahweh his God. He removed the foreign altars and high places, broke down the stone pillars, and cut down the Asherahs. And he commanded Judah to seek Yahweh, the God of their ancestors, and to keep the law and the commandment. And he removed the high places and the incense stands from all the cities of Judah, and the kingdom had rest under him. And he built fortified cities in Judah, for the land was at rest. Under him there was no war in those years, for Yahweh had given rest to him. And he said to Judah, "Let us build these cities and surround them with walls, towers, gates, and bars while the land is before us, because we have sought Yahweh our God. We have sought and he has given rest to us on every side." So they built and had success.

Second Chronicles 14:1–7

THE FIRST TWO rulers of the kingdom of Judah, King Rehoboam and King Abijah, ruled with malevolence, embracing idolatry, defying God's laws, ruthlessly oppressing God's faithful followers, and callously neglecting the welfare of the people (2 Chron. 12:1; 1 Kings 15:3). As King Asa took the throne as the third ruler of Judah, he brought about the long-awaited, very first nationwide religious revival, guided by divine blessing. Under his leadership, the entire nation embraced deep repentance and unwavering resolve, committing resolutely to follow the law and commandments of their God, Yahweh. They purged the land of foreign altars and incense stands dedicated to pagan idol gods that had plagued it for decades. As the Nation of Judah returned to God, divine favor brought a decade of prosperity and peace.

> Asa had an army *of* three hundred thousand from Judah, bearing shields and spears, and two hundred and eighty thousand from Benjamin *who* carried shields and drew bows. All of these *were* mighty warriors of strength. Zerah the Cushite came out against them with an army of a thousand thousands and three hundred chariots. And he came to Mareshah. And Asa went out before him, and a battle was put in order in the valley of Zepah at Mareshah. (2 Chron. 14:8–10)

This decade-long peace in Judah was abruptly disrupted when a massive Cushite army, numbering a million and led by Zerah, attacked Judah's 580,000 soldiers. The Cushite forces also had 300 chariots, while Judah had none.[1] The people of Judah, their hearts pounding with fear, gazed upon the colossal army before them. Despite the overwhelming odds against him, King Asa pressed forward into the battle in the valley of Zepah. With Yahweh, the living God of Israel, surrender was not even in consideration for King Asa of Judah.

---
1 Simon J. De Vries, *1 and 2 Chronicles* (Grand Rapids: Eerdmans, 1989), 299–300.

Then Asa cried out to Yahweh, his God. And he said, "O Yahweh, there is none with you to help between the great and the powerless. Help us, O Yahweh our God, for we rely upon you, and in your name we have come against this multitude. O Yahweh, you *are* our God! Let no man prevail against you!" So Yahweh defeated the Cushites before Asa and before Judah, and the Cushites fled. (2 Chron. 14:11–12)

I *am* Yahweh your God, who brought you out of the land of Egypt, to be your God; I *am* Yahweh your God. (Num. 15:41)

> For I, Yahweh your God, *am* grasping your right hand;
>   *it is I who say* to you,
> "You must not fear;
>   I myself, I will help you."
>
> (Isa. 41:13)

As the army of Judah advanced against the military host of Zerah, King Asa appealed to Yahweh for His intervention. He addressed Yahweh as "our God," meaning the God of Israel. By calling upon this name, he was invoking the covenant God made with the Israelites, where He claimed them as His own. He pleaded with God not to let the enemy prevail over them, for their defeat would be taken as His own. He emphasized that their trust rested solely upon Him, for He is the God of Israel.

The almighty hand of God swept across the battlefield, fortifying the resolve of the Israelites and weakening the Cushites. It was a moment of sheer awe and wonder, a testament to the unmatched power and intervention of God in the face of insurmountable odds. He not only protected His people from the Cushites but also granted them an overwhelming victory.

> Then Asa and the army with him pursued them to Gerar. And *many* from the Cushites fell, for they had no deliverance, for they were shattered before Yahweh and before his army. They carried away much war booty. And they struck all the cities around Gerar, for the fear of Yahweh was upon them. And

they plundered all the cities, for there was much plunder in them. And they also struck the tents of the herdsmen and carried away many sheep and camels. Then they returned to Jerusalem. (2 Chron. 14:13–15)

The Israelites pursued the Cushites to Gerar, which was Philistine territory.[2] They amassed substantial spoils, including a multitude of livestock, from both the Cushites and their Philistine allies. With shouts of joy, they returned to Jerusalem, exulting in Yahweh's complete dominance over the enemy.

> Now Azariah the son of Oded—the Spirit of God came upon him. And he went out before Asa and said to him, "Hear me, O Asa and all of Judah and Benjamin! Yahweh *is* with you while you are with him. If you will seek him he will be found by you. But if you forsake him he will forsake you. Now Israel *has been* without the true God for many days, and without a teaching priest, and without law, but at its trouble he returned to Yahweh, the God of Israel. They sought him, and he was found by them. And in those times, there was no peace for the one going out and the one coming in, for great tumults *were* upon all the inhabitants of the lands. Nation was crushed by nation, and city *was* against city, for God threw them into confusion by all *sorts of* trouble. But as for you, be strong and let not your hands be weak, for there is reward for your labor." (15:1–7)

God sent His prophet Azariah to King Asa while he was still on the road back to Jerusalem following this epic triumph. He intercepted Asa before the jubilant crowds in Jerusalem could sweep him into a celebratory feast, for He had even greater blessings to bestow upon His people. Azariah conveyed that Yahweh had faithfully stood by the Israelites when they sought Him, but their forsaking of Him had led to their abandonment and suffering. He outlined the recurring pattern of disobedience, judgment, suffering, repentance,

---

[2] Heinrich Ewald, *The History of Israel: Vol. IV*, J. Estlin Carpenter, trans. (London: Longmans, Green, and Co., 1878), 50.

and deliverance among His people. To break this vicious cycle, God inspired him to revamp the religious system. The people of Judah needed strong religious leadership to teach them His laws and commandments. God encouraged him to be strong and steadfast in leading this grand revival. God also offered him a reward, which was later revealed as an era of even greater peace and prosperity.

> When Asa heard these words, the prophecy of Oded the prophet, he took courage and removed the vile idols from all the lands of Judah and Benjamin, and from the cities that he had taken in the hill country of Ephraim, and he repaired the altar of Yahweh that was in front of the portico of Yahweh.
>
> And he gathered all Judah and Benjamin and those sojourning with them, from Ephraim, Manasseh, and Simeon, for many had deserted to him from Israel when they saw that Yahweh his God *was* with him. And they were gathered *at* Jerusalem in the third month of the fifteenth year of the reign of Asa. And they sacrificed to Yahweh on that day from the war booty they brought back: seven hundred oxen and seven thousand sheep. And they entered into a covenant to seek Yahweh, the God of their ancestors, with all their heart and with all their inmost being, but all who will not seek Yahweh the God of Israel should be killed, from young to old, from men to women. And they took an oath to Yahweh with a great voice, with shouting, with trumpets, and with horns. And all Judah rejoiced over the oath, for they swore with all their heart. And they sought him with their whole desire, and he was found by them, and Yahweh gave rest to them all around. (2 Chron. 15:8–15)

The living word of God infused King Asa with the courage needed for the grand revival, even in the face of staunch resistance from the elders and nobles in Judah. He purged the land of any remaining pagan idols and began the reconstruction of the Temple of Yahweh. Word of his devotion to God spread, drawing the people of Yahweh from the northern kingdom of Israel. The active force of His words transformed hearts and guided their actions. In a united effort, they gathered in the city of Jerusalem, offering a heartfelt sacrifice to Yahweh. With unyielding determination, they sought His presence, giving every bit of their heart and soul to the pursuit. Just as He had promised Moses 400 years earlier in the wilderness and reaffirmed to Asa on his journey back to Jerusalem, Yahweh came to dwell among them, granting rest, peace, and prosperity (2 Chron. 15:2; Deut. 4:29).

> He said, "You must not fear, O beloved man. *Peace be to you*; be strong and be courageous!" And *when he spoke* with me, I was strengthened and I said, "Let my lord speak, for you have strengthened me." (Dan. 10:19)

> *When he* had said these *things*, he [Jesus] cried out with a loud voice, "Lazarus, come out!" The one who had died came out, his feet and his hands bound with strips of cloth, and his face wrapped with a facecloth. Jesus said to them, "Untie him and let him go." (John 11:43–44)

> Nehemiah the governor, Ezra the priest and scribe, and the Levites who taught the people said to all of the people, "This day is holy to Yahweh your God. Do not mourn nor weep." For all of the people wept when they heard the words of the law. (Neh. 8:9)

> So shall be my word that goes out from my mouth.
>   It shall not return to me without success,
> but shall accomplish what I desire
>   and be successful *in the thing for* which I sent it.
> (Isa. 55:11)

This great revival stands as a testament to the transformative might of God's words, working wonders to accomplish His divine desires. The living words of God are shown in action throughout the Scriptures, fulfilling their divine tasks across different contexts. Through His words, Daniel was strengthened, and Lazarus was brought back from death.

It was also His word that stirred the ardor of true repentance within the hearts of the post-exile generation. They embody the living and active nature of His words, as Yahweh Himself revealed in Isaiah 55:11. The Scriptures also describe the attributes of His words as sharp, piercing, discernible, imperishable, life-giving, instructive, and empowering (Heb. 4:12; 1 Pet. 1:23; John 6:63; 2 Tim. 3:16–17; Matt. 24:35; Ps. 119:89).

> Also Maacah, the mother of Asa, the king removed her from *being* queen, because she had made a repulsive image for Asherah. Asa cut down her repulsive image, and he crushed and burned *it* at the Wadi Kidron. But the high places were not removed from Israel. Nevertheless, the heart of Asa was fully devoted all his days. He brought the holy objects of his father and his own holy objects *into* the house of God—silver and gold and vessels. There was no war until the thirty-fifth year of the reign of Asa. (2 Chron. 15:16–19)

The word "mother" in 15:16 is translated from the Hebrew word *em*, a broad term used to refer to any female ancestor.[3] In this context, it was likely used to denote Maacah as his grandmother, as she gave birth to his father, Abijah (2 Chron. 14:1). King Rehoboam favored Maacah above all his other wives and concubines. He appointed her firstborn, Abijah, as his successor, even though Jeush was the true firstborn (11:18–22).

Through this violation of the Mosaic Law, Maacah rose to the position of *Gebirah* in the kingdom of Judah (Deut. 21:15–17). *Gebirah*, translated as "queen" in 21:16, was an honorable position granted to the mother of the reigning sovereign, with authority over political, religious, and social matters. Maacah likely retained this influential role during Asa's reign due to his mother's early death.[4]

---

3 James E. Smith, *1 & 2 Kings, a Commentary* (n.c., Lulu, 2018), 188–189.

4 Ginny Brewer-Boydston, *Good Queen Mothers, Bad Queen Mothers: The Theological Presentation of the Queen Mother in 1 and 2 Kings* (Eugene, OR: Wipf and Stock, 2023), 89–102.

Maacah's lineage traces back to Tamar, the daughter of Absalom, and her husband, Uriel (1 Chron. 3:2; 2 Chron. 13:2; 1 Kings 15:1–2; 2 Sam. 14:27). Absalom was born to another Maacah, from whom her granddaughter Maacah was named. This earlier Maacah was a princess of Geshur, married to King David (1 Chron. 3:2). Her foreign heritage, stemming from her grandmother, inclined her toward pagan idol worship. She wielded her power to sponsor the cultic activities dedicated to Asherah. Due to the idolatry practice, she was removed from her position of *Gebirah*. With a holy zeal, King Asa shattered and incinerated the Asherah image she made. Following this grand revival, the kingdom of Judah enjoyed a quarter-century of peace and prosperity.

The ABC (Abstract to Brick Concrete)

Revival—General Definition:[5]

- Renewed attention to or interest in something; a new presentation or publication of something old; restoration of force, validity, or effect.

Revival—Biblical Definition:

- A collective process of purging evil and wicked thoughts, feelings, and behaviors within a community, aiming to reestablish a connection with God.

The FAST (Focused, Actionable Steps to Take)

1. Achieving unity is the first step in bringing about revival within a community. Cultivate unity and foster reconciliation within the Christian community, working to resolve conflicts and divisions.

---

5 "Revival," Merriam-Webster.com, accessed October 23, 2023, https://www.merriam-webster.com.

Example: During the Presidential election, a political divide shook the church. Mary stepped up to unite those with differing political affiliations. She emphasized that as followers of Christ, they didn't have to agree on every matter, but they were called to love one another despite their differences (John 13:35). Mary encouraged her fellow church members to shift their focus away from politics and toward their shared faith in Christ.

2. Study Scripture with fellow Christians as a group in pursuit of spiritual renewal and unity. Share devotions to encourage, challenge, and inspire one another.

    Example: Gina took the initiative to bring together her fellow Christians in their church community. Every week, they gather at her house for a Bible study group, where they read and reflect on Scriptures together. Following their study, they share devotions and discussions, deepening their faith and strengthening their sense of community.

19

The Shield of Faith—David

How long, O Yahweh? Will you forget me forever?
How long will you hide your face from me?
How long must I take counsel in my soul,
and sorrow in my heart all the day?
How long will my enemy be exalted over me?
Consider and answer me, O Yahweh my God.
Give light to my eyes lest I sleep the sleep of death,
and lest my enemy should say, "I have overcome him,"
lest my enemies rejoice because I am shaken.

Psalm 13:1–4

In everything tak[e] up the shield of faith, with which you are able to quench all the flaming arrows of the evil one.

Ephesians 6:16

IN PSALM 13, we encounter King David in a state of agonizing waiting for God's deliverance. These repeated cries of "how long" reflect his heartfelt lament over enduring suffering. Every plan he devised to resolve his situation ended in crushing failure, leaving him utterly defeated and his efforts in vain. Those who inflicted the torment only succeeded further.

Amid this misery, he scoured in all directions but found no glint of His deliverance. Desperation led to a haunting fear that God had abandoned him, questioning if the same God who empowered him to conquer Goliath now forsook him. He laid bare his doubts directly before God and asked Him to revive his faith. David knew Yahweh, with His boundless compassion, love, and empathy, would not only forgive his doubts but also revive his faith. He sought to be in His presence, for He is the light that dispels the darkness of doubt.

As written in the book of Ephesians, he understood strong faith serves as a shield against the assaults and temptations of Satan. He feared that the doubts in his heart might lead to separation from God, who Himself is life. This separation would bring a spiritual death, which he aptly referred to as "the sleep of death." The word translated as "shaken" in Psalm 13:4 is the Hebrew term *mot*, denoting a state of profound insecurity.[1] He implores God to restore his faith so he may not be overwhelmed by the relentless pursuit of Satan.

> But as for me, I have trusted in your steadfast love.
> My heart will rejoice in your deliverance.
> I will sing to Yahweh
> because he has dealt bountifully with me.
>
> (13:5–6)

Now if you will carefully listen to my voice and keep my covenant, you will be a treasured possession for me out of all the peoples, *for all the earth is mine*. . . . Moses wrote all the words of Yahweh, and he rose early in the morning, and he built an altar at the base of the mountain and *set up* twelve memorial stones for the twelve tribes of Israel. . . . He took the scroll of the

---

1 John D. Barry, et al., eds., *NKJV Faithlife Illustrated Study Bible* (Grand Rapids: Zondervan, 2018), 858.

covenant and read *it* in the hearing of the people, and they said, "All that Yahweh has spoken we will do, and we will listen." And Moses took the blood and sprinkled *it* on the people, and he said, "Look, the blood of the covenant that Yahweh has made with you in accordance with all these words." (Exod. 19:5; 24:4, 7–8)

In Psalm 13:5, the phrase "steadfast love" originates from the Hebrew word *hesed*, which conveys the idea of covenantal love.[2] This represents His fiercely loyal affection for His chosen people, as established in the covenant recorded in Exodus chapters 19 to 24.[3] In the latter part of the psalm, Yahweh answers his prayer with His comforting presence. David undergoes a deep spiritual revival, with his faith, hope, and joy abundantly renewed. David offers a song of praise to Yahweh for His unwavering faithfulness in this graceful restoration.

The ABC (Abstract to Brick Concrete)

Faith—General Definition:[4]

- Allegiance to duty or a person; belief and trust in and loyalty to God; firm belief in something for which there is no proof; something that is believed especially with strong conviction.

Faith—Biblical Definition:

- The unwavering trust and belief in God's sacred covenants and divine characteristics, shielding Christians from temptations and deceit.

---

2 Steven J. Lawson, *Psalms 1–75* (Brentwood, TN: B&H Publishing Group, 2003), 72–73.

3 Gerald Henry Wilson, *The NIV Application Commentary: Psalms—Volume 1* (Grand Rapids: Zondervan, 2002), 400–401.

4 "Faith," Merriam-Webster.com, accessed October 23, 2023, https://www.merriam-webster.com.

The FAST (Focused, Actionable Steps to Take)

In the book of Romans, the apostle Paul emphasized that faith grows through studying God's Word (Rom. 10:17). Therefore, it is important for us to regularly study the Scriptures to continually strengthen our faith.

Example 1: Wendy's daily practice of immersing herself in God's Word and prayer protected her when exposed to a false doctrine by a church friend. Her well-grounded faith enabled her to recognize the error, question it, and gently guide her friend back to the genuine teachings of the Bible. Her faith served as a protective shield against the deceit, reinforcing that faith is a powerful defense against spiritual challenges.

Example 2: Brian's daily scripture study deepens his faith and shields him from the temptation of gambling. He once struggled with this vice but, through regular scripture reflection, found strength in biblical teachings that emphasized self-control and responsible stewardship. His faith, nurtured by Scripture, empowered him to overcome the temptation and make positive changes in his life.

20

The Repurposed— Jeremiah

The words of Jeremiah, the son of Hilkiah, among the priests who were *in Anathoth, in the land of Benjamin,* to *whom the word of Yahweh came in the days of Josiah the son of Amon, the king of Judah, in the thirteenth year of his reign. It came also in the days of Jehoiakim, the son of Josiah, the king of Judah, until the end of the eleventh year of Zedekiah, the son of Josiah, the king of Judah, until the exile of Jerusalem in the fifth month. And the word of Yahweh came to me,* saying, *"Before I formed you in the womb I knew you, and before you came out from* the *womb I consecrated you; I appointed you* as *a prophet to the nations." Then I said, "Ah, Lord Yahweh! Look, I do not know* how *to speak, for I* am *a youth."*

Jeremiah 1:1–6

ANATHOTH WAS one of the four cities in the land of Benjamin allocated to the Levites, who held the role of priests (Josh. 21:8, 17–18). This city was often referred to as a "storehouse," as it absorbed northern influences from Bethel, located eight miles away, and southern traditions from Jerusalem, situated just three miles down the road.[1] Jeremiah grew up in this priestly town, where he followed in his father's footsteps and received training to carry on his family's tradition of priesthood. However, his life took an unexpected turn when Yahweh revealed Himself to him and appointed him as His prophet. This was unusual because, during that time, prophets were typically trained in schools of prophets. Prophets who graduated from schools of prophets typically received support from them when facing resistance from the elders and nobles of the kingdom of Judah or the Temple priests. This support system provided protection and assistance, which Jeremiah lacked as he had not attended such a school.[2]

In response to the divine calling, Jeremiah tells God that he does not know how to speak because he is a youth. The word Jeremiah used to describe himself, "youth," is derived from the Hebrew word *naar*. *Naar* is a versatile term that can mean youthful, inexperienced, unproven, or signify the status of a servant, student, or trainee.[3] In this context, he likely used this term to express his lack of education, training for the role of a prophet, and overall qualifications for the work. It suggests that he felt ill-prepared and inexperienced for the prophetic role, akin to a classic pianist unexpectedly transitioning to become a keyboard player for a rock and roll concert.

---

1 Robert Chazan, William W. Hallo, and Lawrence H. Schiffman, eds., *Ki Baruch Hu: Ancient Near Eastern, Biblical, and Judaic Studies in Honor of Baruch A. Levine* (Winona Lake, IN: Eisenbrauns, 1999), 264–266.

2 J.R. Gillies, *Jeremiah The Man and His Message* (London: Hodder and Stoughton, 1907), 180–181.

3 Matityahu Clark and Samson Raphael Hirsch, *Etymological Dictionary of Biblical Hebrew: Based on the Commentaries of Rabbi Samson Raphael Hirsch* (Nanuet, NY: Feldheim Publishers, 1999), 159.

But Yahweh said to me, "You must not say, 'I *am* a youth,' for to *whomever* I send you, you will go, and *whatever* I command you, you will speak. *Do not be afraid of them*, for I *am* with you to deliver you," *declares* Yahweh. Then Yahweh stretched out his hand and he touched my mouth, and Yahweh said to me,

> "Look, I have put my words in your mouth.
> See, I appoint you this day over the nations
> and over the kingdoms,
> to pluck up and to pull down,
> and to destroy and to tear down,
> to build and to plant."

> And the word of Yahweh came to me, *saying*, "What *are* you seeing, Jeremiah?" And I said, "I *am* seeing a branch of an almond tree." Then Yahweh said to me, "You did well to see, for I *am* watching over my word to perform it." (Jer. 1:7–12)

Yahweh stretched out His hand and touched Jeremiah's mouth. With this divine touch, he became equipped with the power to articulate with authority, dignity, and eloquence. Yaweh then showed Jeremiah a branch of an almond tree, which is *saqed* in Hebrew. The word *saqed* is derived from *saqad*, meaning "to watch or to wake." This almond tree is aptly named the "awake tree" because it is the first tree to bud and bear fruit in the year. Its blossoms appear before its leaves as the tree bursts into bloom in January.[4] God employed this vision of an almond tree as a wordplay to symbolize the unshakable sovereignty in fulfilling His words.

> The word of Yahweh came to me a second *time, saying*, "What *are* you seeing?" And I said, "I *am* seeing a *boiling* pot, and its face *is* from *the* face of *the* north." Then Yahweh said to me, "From *the* north disaster will be unleashed on all the inhabitants of the land. For, look, I *am* calling to all *the* clans of *the*

---

4 John F. Walvoord and Roy B. Zuck, *Bible Knowledge Commentary: Old Testament* (Colorado Springs: David C. Cook, 1985), 1131–1132.

kingdoms of *the* north," *declares* Yahweh, "and they will come and set each one his throne *at* the entrance of the gates of Jerusalem, and against all its surrounding walls, and against all the cities of Judah. And I will pass my judgments on them because of all their wickedness *in* that they have forsaken me, and they made sacrifices to other gods, and they bowed in worship to the works of their hands." (Jer. 1:13–16)

God granted Jeremiah a second vision—a turbulent boiling pot teetering from north to south, its contents nearly overflowing. This symbolized the impending disaster on Judah, akin to the scalding spill from a boiling pot. While Babylonia was east of Judah geographically, its armies opted not to cross the harsh Arabian desert. Instead, they followed the Euphrates River northward into Syria and invaded Judah from the north.[5] This vision alluded to His plan to employ their enemy as an instrument of judgment upon the kingdom of Judah.

"But you, you must gird your loins, and stand, and speak to them all that I command you. *Do not be afraid of them*, or I will shatter you *before* them. Now look, I have made you *today* as a fortified city and as an iron pillar and a bronze wall against all the land, against the kings of Judah, against its princes, against its priests, and against the people of the land. And they will fight against you but they will not prevail against you, for I *am* with you," *declares* Yahweh, "to deliver you." (1:17–19)

When God instructed Jeremiah to gird up his loins, it was akin to a call for immediate preparedness and readiness for action. During those times, individuals wore lengthy robes that could hinder swift movement. The act of girding up one's loins involved securing the lower part of the robe around the waist, effectively facilitating mobility. This practice can be likened to

---

[5] F.B. Huey, *Jeremiah, Lamentations: An Exegetical and Theological Exposition of Holy Scripture* (Nashville: Broadman, 1993), 54.

the modern notion of rolling up one's sleeves before embarking on a task.[6]

God commanded His prophet not to fear the people, for he would only be forsaken, thus "shattered," if he succumbed to fear and listened to them instead of obeying Him. He reassured Jeremiah that He would stand by his side as he delivered the messages of divine judgment to the nation. He promised to protect Jeremiah from anyone who opposed him for proclaiming His words.

Jeremiah's life exemplifies how a calling from God can divert from personal desires and societal norms. His divine purpose as a prophet was not what he might have imagined or what society expected of him. Yet, in this unexpected calling, God equipped him with extraordinary courage, unwavering strength, and the endurance needed to fulfill his mission. This divine preparation didn't require years of training at a prophet school; it came with the calling itself, providing all he would need to fulfill his extraordinary mission.

The ABC (Abstract to Brick Concrete)

Calling—General Definition:[7]

- A strong inner impulse toward a particular course of action; the vocation or profession in which one customarily engages.

Calling—Biblical Definition:

- God's intended purpose of creation for the individual, accompanied by divine authority, guidance, and all the necessary attributes and provisions required to fulfill the assigned duty.

---

6 Huey, 56.

7 "Calling," Merriam-Webster.com, accessed October 23, 2023, https://www.merriam-webster.com.

The FAST (Focused, Actionable Steps to Take)

While each of us has our own unique calling, together, we are all called to be followers of Christ and to be faithful to our calling to spread the gospel to people of all nations (Matt. 28:18–20).

Example 1: Darlene uses her social media platforms to share daily Scripture, devotionals, and encouraging messages with a global audience. Every morning, she selects a Bible verse and crafts a related devotional to inspire her followers. Her engaging content fosters a digital community where diverse individuals find solace, hope, and spiritual guidance. She actively interacts with them, offering support, answering questions, and engaging in meaningful conversations about the gospel.

Example 2: Every Sunday, right after church, Christine and a group of church members head downtown to hand out Christian pamphlets on the gospel. They set up near a bustling intersection, offering pamphlets filled with messages of hope and salvation to people passing by. With friendly smiles and personal stories of their own faith, they connect with individuals from different backgrounds, sharing the gospel.

21

Faith in the Fire—Peter

Peter, an apostle of Jesus Christ, to the chosen who are residing temporarily in the dispersion in Pontus, Galatia, Cappadocia, Asia, and Bithynia, according to the foreknowledge of God the Father, by the sanctification of the Spirit, for obedience and **for** *sprinkling with the blood of Jesus Christ. May grace and peace be multiplied to you.*

First Peter 1:1–2

THE APOSTLE PETER addresses his letter to "the chosen ones" who are temporarily residing in the dispersion across a vast area of the central and northern plateau of Asia Minor, which corresponds to the modern nation of Turkey.[1] "The chosen ones" in this context are followers of Christ scattered among unbelievers. They were selected by God the Father through the work of the Spirit to partake in the new covenant established by Christ's blood. Their way of life and relationships shifted in alignment with the teachings of Christ, causing them to become sojourners in society.[2]

---

1 Paul A. Himes, *Foreknowledge and Social Identity in 1 Peter* (Eugene, OR: Wipf and Stock, 2014), 132.
2 Karen H. Jobes, *1 Peter (Baker Exegetical Commentary on the New Testament)*, 2nd ed. (Grand Rapids: Baker Academic, 2005, 2022), 63–80.

> Blessed *be* the God and Father of our Lord Jesus Christ, who according to his great mercy has caused us to be born again to a living hope through the resurrection of Jesus Christ from the dead, into an inheritance imperishable and undefiled and unfading, reserved in heaven for you who are being protected by the power of God through faith for a salvation ready to be revealed in the last time, in which you rejoice greatly, *although* now for a short time, if necessary, you are distressed by various trials, so that the genuineness of your faith, more valuable than gold that is passing away, but is tested by fire, may be found to *result in* praise and glory and honor at the revelation of Jesus Christ, whom, *although you* have not seen, you love; in whom now you believe, *although you* do not see *him*, and you rejoice greatly with joy inexpressible and full of glory, obtaining the goal of your faith, the salvation of *your* souls. (1 Pet. 1:3–9)

Peter reminds Christians of their rebirth and salvation through their faith in Christ. He compares the trials they may encounter to the process of refining gold through fire, urging them to see these challenges as stepping stones on their path to spiritual maturity rather than as obstacles. He emphasizes that these trials will strengthen their faith, making it unshakable and deserving of praise from Christ. Peter encourages them to fix their gaze on the eternal heavenly home and the imperishable inheritance awaiting their arrival. These profound insights serve as a guiding light for Christians, enabling them to steadfastly endure the weighty trials of this world as they recognize that these challenges are integral steps on their path to spiritual growth and the promise of a more glorious destination in heaven.

> Concerning this salvation, the prophets who prophesied about the grace meant for you sought and made careful inquiry, investigating for what *person* or which time the Spirit of Christ in them was indicating *when he* testified beforehand to the sufferings with reference to Christ and the glories after these *things*, to whom it was revealed that they were serving not themselves

but you with reference to the same *things* which now have been announced to you through those who proclaimed the gospel to you by the Holy Spirit sent from heaven, *things into which* angels desire to look. Therefore, *when you have prepared your minds for action by* being self-controlled, put your hope completely in the grace that will be brought to you at the revelation of Jesus Christ. (1 Pet. 1:10–13)

Peter then explains that the prophets who foretold Christ's suffering and glory were eager to understand when and for whom these revelations were meant. Even the angels shared this eagerness for understanding. Peter emphasizes that this truth constitutes the gospel, empowered by the Holy Spirit.

He underscores the importance of self-control in preparing one's mind to follow closely in the footsteps of Christ. In 1:13, the Greek word for "self-control" is *nephontes*, conveying full attentiveness and sobriety.[3] It is important to differentiate this from *egkrateia*, translated as "self-control" in Galatians 5:23. This Greek word *egkrateia* represents the virtue of mastering desires and passions.[4]

> As obedient children, do not be conformed to the former desires *you used to conform to* in your ignorance, but as the one who called you *is* holy, *you* yourselves be holy in all *your* conduct, for it is written, "You will be holy, because I *am* holy." And if you call on *him as* Father who judges impartially according to each one's work, conduct yourselves with fear during the time of your temporary residence, *because you* know that you were redeemed from your futile way of life inherited from your ancestors not with perishable things like silver or gold, but with the precious blood of Christ, like *that of* an unblemished and spotless lamb who was foreknown before the foundation of the world, but has been revealed in these last times for you who through him *are*

---

3 J. Ramsey Michaels, *1 Peter, Volume 49* (Grand Rapids: Zondervan Academic, 2015), 55.

4 Bruce B. Barton, et al., eds., *1&2 Peter and Jude: Life Application Bible Commentary* 1995), 166.

believing in God, who raised him from the dead and gave him glory, so that your faith and hope are in God. (1 Pet. 1:14–21)

Peter cites Leviticus 19:2 to underscore the idea that because God is holy, nothing unholy can stand before Him. This is why God called His chosen people to be holy, allowing them to maintain a close relationship with Him. Peter extends this divine call to Christians, encouraging them to lead lives that set them apart while living in the secular society they are scattered in, all to stay united with Christ.

In their earthly existence, Peter instructs the believers to maintain a sense of awe and reverence toward God, living in a manner that reflects their distinctiveness from the worldly desires they once followed in their ignorance. This transformation toward holiness and fear of God would allow them to walk with Him throughout their lives.

Christians have been redeemed from a life in which they toiled relentlessly for perishable things, only to leave this world empty-handed after all their efforts. They now work for Christ, who rewards them with blessings that extend into eternity (John 6:26–27). Peter highlights that this redemption was not achieved through worldly wealth like silver or gold but through the precious blood of Christ. His plan to redeem the chosen ones through His own blood preceded the very creation of the world.

> Having purified your souls by your obedience to the truth for sincere brotherly love, love one another fervently from the heart, *because you* have been born again, not from a perishable seed but imperishable, through the living and enduring word of God. For
>
> > "all flesh *is* like grass,
> > and all its glory is like the flower of the grass.
> > The grass withers and the flower falls off,
> > but the word of the Lord endures *forever*."
>
> And this is the word that has been proclaimed to you. (1 Pet. 1:22–25)

In First Peter 1:22, the word "fervently" springs from the Greek word *ektenos*, which has its roots in a medical term for stretching a muscle to its absolute limit, much like what athletes do when pushing their physical boundaries.[5] Peter uses this athletic imagery to illustrate a point. Just as athletes stretch their muscles to their utmost capacity, he urges Christians to put their wholehearted dedication into loving one another. This teaching echoes the words of Christ, a new commandment for us to love one another as He has loved us (John 13:34–35). Peter urges them to align their way of life and relationships with the teachings of Christ because they have been born again "through the living and enduring word of God," which is Christ Himself. He quotes Isaiah (40:6, 8), in which Christ is referred to as the Word of God, to emphasize His eternal and everlasting nature. Peter's reference to Christ as the Word of God is not isolated; it is a statement that finds resonance with the apostle John throughout the Scriptures (John 1:1–5; Rev. 19:11–13).

The ABC (Abstract to Brick Concrete)

Trial—General Definition:[6]

- The action of putting to the proof; a tryout or experiment to test quality, value, or usefulness; a test of faith, patience, or stamina through subjection to suffering or temptation.

Trial—Biblical Definition:

- A challenging experience that tests one's faith, making it stronger as the individuals prepare themselves for eternal life in heaven.

---

5 John H. Hill, *Peter's Epistles: Letters to the Scattered Saints*. (n.c., Lulu [self-published], 2019), 142.

6 Trial," Merriam-Webster.com, accessed October 23, 2023, https://www.merriam-webster.com.

The FAST (Focused, Actionable Steps to Take)

When confronted with a trial, place your hope and faith in Christ rather than relying on wealth, social status, or other people.

Example: After suffering a stroke that left him unable to walk, Martin, a recovering alcoholic, demonstrated unwavering resilience. Instead of returning to alcohol, he relied on his faith in Christ. Martin engaged in daily prayer, read Scripture, and became an active member of his church community for support. He shared his story to inspire others and practiced gratitude and forgiveness. In doing so, Martin persevered, remaining sober and growing spiritually.

22

A Little Leaven Leavens the Whole Batch of Dough—Jude

Jude, a slave of Jesus Christ and brother of James, to **those who are** *called, loved in God the Father and kept for Jesus Christ. May mercy and peace and love be multiplied to you. Dear friends,* **although** *I was making every effort to write to you concerning our common salvation, I considered* **it** *a necessity to write to you to encourage* **you** *to contend for the faith delivered once and for all to the saints. For certain men have slipped in stealthily, who were designated long ago for this condemnation, ungodly ones, who change the grace of our God into licentiousness and who deny our only Master and Lord Jesus Christ.*

Jude 1–4

JUDE, THE HALF-BROTHER of Jesus (and the full brother of James the Just), chose not to lean on his familial connection with Jesus. Instead, he humbly identified himself as His slave. This humility and lack of self-promotion emerged from his deep recognition of Jesus as the Christ. Right from the outset, he clearly states the purpose of his letter is to alert fellow Christians to those who promote false doctrines and lead others astray. These false teachers become recognizable by their disregard for God, denial of Christ, and distortion of God's grace to justify further sinful conduct.

> Now I want to remind you, *although* you know everything once and for all, that Jesus, having saved the people out of the land of Egypt, the second time destroyed those who did not believe. And *the* angels who did not keep to their own domain but deserted their proper dwelling place, he has kept in eternal bonds under deep gloom for the judgment of the great day, as Sodom and Gomorrah and the towns around them indulged in sexual immorality and *pursued unnatural desire in* the same way as these, are exhibited as an example *by* undergoing the punishment of eternal fire. Despite that, in the same way also these *men, because of their* dreams, defile the flesh and reject authority and blaspheme majestic beings. (Jude 5–8)

> He [Christ] ordered them [His disciples], saying, "Watch out! Beware of the leaven of the Pharisees and the leaven of Herod!" (Mark 8:15)

> Your boasting *is* not good. Do you not know that a little leaven leavens the whole batch of dough? Clean out the old leaven in order that you may be a new batch of dough, just as you are unleavened. For Christ our Passover has been sacrificed. So then, let us celebrate the feast, not with the old leaven or with the leaven of wickedness and sinfulness, but with the unleavened bread of sincerity and truth. (1 Cor. 5:6–8)

Jude offers examples of divine judgment for those who practice false doctrines and lead others astray. The first case involves the Israelites who returned from surveying the promised land with mistrust toward God. This unbelief spread among the community, leading to the death of that entire generation, except for Joshua and Caleb, who remained faithful (Num. 14:2, 22–24). Jude then discusses the angels who abandoned their assigned duties, rebelling against God and corrupting other angels, leading to their imprisonment in darkness.[1] Finally, he mentions the people of Sodom and Gomorrah, whose sinful rebellion extended to neighboring nations and ultimately perished in heavenly fire (Gen. 19:24–25).

Due to the pervasive nature of leaven, there is a saying: "A little leaven leavens the whole batch of dough." Christ employed leaven as a symbol for harmful doctrines that can corrupt the entire community. Examples of the leaven of wickedness and sin include the generation of unbelief and disobedience in the wilderness, the angels who rebelled to elevate themselves, and the sinful people of Sodom and Gomorrah. God removed the leaven to preserve holiness among His chosen ones, represented by the unleavened bread of truth. Jude forewarns that false shepherds will ultimately face divine condemnation and punishment.

Jude highlights how people can be misled by false dreamers (Jude 8). This observation is not limited to Jude, as Moses, Jeremiah, and Zechariah also addressed such dreamers in their respective times (Deut. 13:1–3; Jer. 27:9–10; Zech. 10:2).

> But Michael the archangel, when he argued with the devil, disputing concerning the body of Moses, did not dare to pronounce a blasphemous judgment, but said, "The Lord rebuke you!" But these persons blaspheme all that they do not understand, and all that they understand by instinct like the irrational animals, by these *things* they are being destroyed. Woe to them! For they have traveled in the way of Cain, and have given themselves up to the error of Balaam for gain, and have perished in the rebellion of Korah. These are the ones feasting together without reverence, hidden reefs at your love feasts, caring for themselves, waterless clouds carried away by winds, late autumn trees without fruit, twice dead, uprooted,

---

1 Randal S. Chase, *New Testament Study Guide, Pt. 3: The Epistles and Book of Revelation* (Washington, UT: Plain & Precious Publishing, 2010), 318–319.

wild waves of the sea foaming up their own shameful deeds, wandering stars, for whom the deep gloom of darkness has been reserved for eternity. (Jude 9–13)

Then Joseph said to them [his brothers], "Do not be afraid, for *am* I in the place of God?" (Gen. 50:19)

Jude employs the example of the archangel Michael to emphasize the divine sovereignty in judgment and punishment. In his role, Michael abstains from personal judgments and punishments, entrusting these matters solely to God's hands.[2] Another powerful example comes from the story of Joseph in the book of Genesis. In reply to his brothers' plea for forgiveness, Joseph humbly stated he lacked the authority to judge or punish them. He pointed out that such matters rest solely in the hands of God. Jude emphasizes that in stark contrast to the earlier mentioned examples, the heretics engage in harsh judgments and punitive actions despite their lack of understanding of sound doctrine.

He reveals that followers of apostasy are driven by three primary motives: sin and wickedness, like Cain; a pursuit of earthly wealth, like Balaam; and a thirst for power, like Korah. Their misguided faith exposes itself through greed, particularly during love feasts where they selfishly consume food meant for the poor. Their grandiose claims are not followed through, akin to rainless clouds and fruitless trees. With their confident speeches, they appear to carry all before them, but like waves crashing upon the shore, their impact dissipates, leaving only their shame. Jude calls the followers of false teaching as "twice dead" to illustrate the initial death to self through their spiritual rebirth in Christ, followed by a subsequent state of spiritual death resulting from their apostasy.

Enoch, the seventh from Adam, also prophesied about these *people*, saying, "Behold, the Lord came with tens of thousands of his holy ones to execute judgment against all, and to convict all the ungodly concerning all their ungodly deeds that they

---
2 Chase, 318–319.

have committed in an ungodly way, and concerning all the harsh things that ungodly sinners have spoken against him. These *people* are grumblers, discontented, proceeding according to their desires, and their mouths speaking pompous *words, showing partiality to gain an advantage.*

But you, dear friends, remember the words proclaimed beforehand by the apostles of our Lord Jesus Christ, for they said to you, "In the end time there will be scoffers following according to their own ungodly desires." These are the ones who cause divisions, worldly, not having the Spirit. But you, dear friends, *by* building yourselves up in your most holy faith, *by* praying in the Holy Spirit, keep yourselves in the love of God, looking forward to the mercy of our Lord Jesus Christ to eternal life. And have mercy on those who doubt, and save others *by* snatching *them* from the fire, and have mercy on others with fear, hating even the tunic stained by the flesh. (Jude 14–23)

Jude references a passage from First Enoch that describes the second coming of Christ as a judgment upon the world.[3]

He characterizes "the ungodly" on whom the punishment will fall as grumbling, discontent, selfish, arrogant, and unjust. In verse 16, "grumbler" is translated from the Greek word *goggustes*, which implies muttered expressions filled with disdain and resentment. This term is onomatopoeic, resembling the cooing of doves.[4] In Hebrew, its counterpart is *lun*, derived from the sound camels make when refusing to move—a willful disobedience. This word encompasses more than mere grumbling; it includes stubbornly remaining behind and refusing to proceed forward.[5]

---

[3] First Enoch 1:9. (First Enoch is one of several noncanonical books known as the Pseudepigrapha.)

[4] Guy Manuell, *The Letter of Jude: A Wake-Up Call to Christians in the Twenty-First Century* (Bloomington, IN: Westbow Press, 2022), 42, 161–163.

[5] R. Alan Cole, *Exodus, Tyndale Old Testament Commentaries* (Downers Grove, IL: Inter-Varsity Press, 1973), 128.

The Israelites who grumbled against God were denied entry into the promised land, resulting in their deaths in the wilderness (Num. 14:2, 22–24). Jude highlights the sin of harboring disdain and resentment toward God and how it leads to disobedience, which would similarly hinder their entry into His kingdom. The word "discontented" in Jude 16 was translated from the Greek term *mempsimoiros*, which points to a perpetual fault-finder blaming their own fate throughout life rather than being discontent due to a particular issue.[6] Cultivating gratitude and contentment honors the divine and also instills a sense of humility. These virtues serve as the groundwork of the path to God's kingdom, preparing the heart to receive His abundant grace and mercy.

Jude highlights scoffers as responsible for divisions within the congregation. These individuals may appear Christian, but their worldly desires have led them astray. They initially experienced a spiritual rebirth through Christ but later succumbed to worldly desires. Despite their familiarity with the gospels and sound doctrine, they now mock these teachings instead of following them, having lost their reverence for God. Such scoffers serve as indicators that the second coming of Christ is drawing near.

In preparation for judgment day, Jude provides practical strategies to avoid sharing the fate of those facing punishment. These strategies encompass living in accordance with one's faith, studying and following God's word, seeking guidance in prayer from the Holy Spirit, demonstrating love for God and fellow Christians, and placing hope in Christ for salvation and eternal life.

> Now to the one who is able to protect you from stumbling and make *you* to stand before his glory blameless with exultation, to the only God our Savior, through Jesus Christ our Lord, *be* glory, majesty, power, and authority before all time and now and for all eternity. Amen. (Jude 24–25)

---

6 John H. Hill, *Jude - Epistle of Identification* (n.c., Lulu, 2011), 101.

With His everlasting reign, the teachings of Christ remain eternally true. Jude closes his letter by praising Christ for His sovereign power to protect believers from falling into the false teachings mentioned earlier.

The ABC (Abstract to Brick Concrete)

Apostasy—General Definition:[7]

- An act of refusing to continue to follow, obey, or recognize a religious faith; abandonment of a previous loyalty

Apostasy—Biblical Definition:

- A misleading belief system characterized by disregard for God, denial of Christ, and the distortion of religious principles, often used to justify sinful behavior

The FAST (Focused, Actionable Steps to Take)

Stay alert for individuals promoting deceitful teachings that involve the denial of Christ.

Example: Mercedes was attending a fellowship gathering one evening when she noticed an individual promoting a false doctrine denying the true deity of Christ. Troubled by what she heard, she consulted her senior pastor, Pastor Luke, who appreciated her vigilance in protecting the church's faith. They discussed how to best address the issue with wisdom and compassion, praying for discernment. With Mercedes' diligence and the support of Pastor Luke, the church took steps to address the issue, ensuring that the congregation remained firmly grounded in their faith and protected from the influence of the false doctrine.

---

7 "Apostasy," Merriam-Webster.com, accessed October 23, 2023, https://www.merriam-webster.com.

23

Guided by the Fear of God

Send out your bread on the water, for in many days you will find it. Divide your share in seven or eight, for you do not know what disaster will happen on the earth. When the clouds are full, they empty rain on the earth. Whether a tree falls to the south or whether it falls to the north, the place where the tree falls—there it will be. Whoever watches the wind will not sow; whoever watches the clouds will not reap. Just as you do not know how the path of the wind goes, nor how the bones of a fetus form in a mother's womb, so you do not know the work of God who makes everything. Sow your seed in the morning, and do not let your hands rest in the evening, for you do not know what will prosper— whether this or that, or whether both of them alike will succeed.

Ecclesiastes 11:1–6

Ask rain from Yahweh in the season of the spring rain— Yahweh, who makes storm clouds, and he gives showers of rain to them, to everyone vegetation in the field.

Zechariah 10:1

THE PREACHER OPENS his speech by imploring people to send their bread out on the water. In his time, many of the poor toiled on long voyages aboard commercial trading ships. This was the preacher's way of telling them to give their material possessions to those in need, including the poor who went to sea.[1] Although this act may seem like a waste of bread, his message is that they will receive their reward in the future, both in this world and in the world to come. In essence, it encourages taking action now for rewards that may not be immediately apparent.

He advises diversifying efforts because it is impossible to foresee which might fail. This advice aligns with the American saying "Don't put all your eggs in one basket," which means to avoid concentrating all efforts and resources in one place to avoid a catastrophic loss.

He describes factors beyond human control that can unexpectedly lead to the failure of their efforts. For example, he mentions weather conditions, subject to divine sovereignty, as described in Zechariah 10:1. He illustrates how humans cannot even dictate the direction in which a tree will fall, underscoring the limitations of human endeavors.

The preacher advises people to work diligently throughout the day, noting that early efforts may not yield immediately visible results. He urges them to place their hope in Yahweh because worldly pursuits such as wealth and power are as fleeting as the wind and clouds, offering no lasting rewards.

> The light is sweet,
> > and it *is* pleasant for the eyes to see the sun.
> For if a man lives many years,
> > let him rejoice in all of them!
> Let him remember that the days of the darkness will be many—
> > all that is coming *is* vanity!

---

[1] Aramaic Targum to Ecclesiastes 11:1, https://www.sefaria.org/Aramaic_Targum_to_Ecclesiastes.

> Rejoice, O young man, in your youth,
>   and let your heart cheer you in the days of your youth!
> Follow the ways of your heart and the sight of your eyes—
>   but know that God will bring you into judgment for all these things.
> Banish anxiety from your heart,
>   and put away pain from your body,
> for youth and vigor *are* vanity.
>
> (Eccles. 11:7–10)

God said, "Let there be light!" And there was light. God saw the light, that *it was* good, and God caused *there to be* a separation between the light and between the darkness. (Gen. 1:3–4)

> He who is steadfast in righteousness *is* to life
>   as he who pursues evil *is* to death.
>
> (Prov. 11:19)

The Hebrew term *towb* is translated as "pleasant" in Ecclesiastes 11:7 and "good" in Genesis 1:4. *Towb* essentially means goodness in its broadest sense, signifying perfection. Both Genesis 1:4 and Ecclesiastes 11:7 celebrate the divine goodness of God, symbolized as the sun in 11:7.[2]

His light is also referred to as "sweet," a translation from the Hebrew word *mathoq*. This term conveys the gustatory sensation of detecting a flavor akin to honey.[3] The presence of God is not only illuminating but also brings a profound sense of delight and comfort, similar to the pleasurable sweetness of honey to the taste.

The preacher cleverly deploys sarcasm as a teaching method for young individuals. His words seemingly advise them to pursue their worldly desires but are actually delivered with a

---

2 Muhammad Wolfgang G.A. Schmidt, *A Hebrew-English Reference Manual To The Hebrew Text Of The Old Testament* (Hamburg, Germany: disserta Verlag, 2017), 226.

3 J.D. Douglas, Moises Silva, and Merrill Chapin Tenney, *Zondervan Illustrated Bible Dictionary* (Grand Rapids: Zondervan, 2011), 961.

touch of irony. It's his way of rhetorically cautioning against the pursuit of secular desires. He earnestly warns them of the divine judgment that awaits them at the end of their earthly lives for all their actions.

In Ecclesiastes 11:10, the term "anxiety" is translated from the Hebrew word *kaas*, which can also be translated as vexation, provocation, causing anger, deeply frustrating, and exasperating in English. It refers to the tendency to engage in repetitive and persistently irritating actions or behaviors.[4] An example of such actions would be persistently provoking an individual until it triggers their anger. The preacher advises people to eliminate such inclinations since they often lead to malevolent or wicked behaviors.

The term "pain" in 11:10 comes from the Hebrew word *raah*, which can also be translated as evil, wickedness, bad, ungodly, misery, or disaster in English. This word is the most common antonym to *towb*, signifying perfection, righteousness, and godliness.[5] "Righteousness" and "evil" in Proverbs 11:19 are translated from *towb* and *raah*, respectively. The preacher counsels them to abstain from evil actions, particularly during one's fleeting youth.

He counsels the people to live with a fear of God, emphasizing that divine judgments await them at the end of their lives. He paints a picture of human life on Earth as a transient journey, likening people to sojourners. Taking a broader view, he underscores that in eternity, the only thing that truly holds significance is a faithful life lived for the glory of God, which God graciously rewards with enduring blessings.

---

4 Isaac Landman and Simon Cohen, *The Universal Jewish Encyclopedia: An Authoritative and Popular Presentation of Jews and Judaism Since the Earliest Times* (New York: Universal Jewish Encyclopedia, Inc., 1943). 314–316.

5 Kari Storstein Haug, *Interpreting Proverbs 11:18–31, Psalm 73, and Ecclesiastes 9:1–12 in Light of, and as a Response to, Thai Buddhist Interpretations* (Leiden, The Netherlands: Brill, 2012), 192–194.

The ABC (Abstract to Brick Concrete)

Reverence—General Definition:[6]

- Honor or respect felt or shown; regarded as worthy.

Reverence—Biblical Definition:

- The fear of God, rooted in the belief in divine judgments, where the faithful are met with eternal blessings, and the evil receive lasting punishment.

The FAST (Focused, Actionable Steps to Take)

Live with the fear of God, knowing that living faithfully and doing good deeds for the glory of God leads to eternal blessings, while a wicked life of evil deeds results in lasting punishment.

Example: David lives with the fear of God, consistently choosing good over evil by adhering to the teachings of Christ in the Bible. He aims to lead a life that reflects the love, compassion, and integrity demonstrated by Christ.

---

6 "Reverence," Merriam-Webster.com, accessed October 23, 2023, https://www.merriam-webster.com.

24

Singing Under the Stars—The Levites

Look, bless Yahweh, all you *the servants of Yahweh, who* serve *in the house of Yahweh by night. Lift up your hands in* the *sanctuary and bless Yahweh. May Yahweh bless you from Zion,* he who *made heaven and earth.*

Psalm 134:1–3

Some of the Levites were *scribes, officials, and gatekeepers.*

Second Chronicles 34:13

Now these were *the singers; the heads of the* families *of the Levites* were *in the chambers free from other service, for day and night* they were *over them on the service.*

First Chronicles 9:33

PSALM 134 STANDS out as a nighttime song of praise performed by the Levites. They were the sole individuals occupying the Temple service during the night, serving as either singers or gatekeepers.[1] As the night deepened, their voices rose in a harmonious chorus, and their words became a song. Lifting their hands in unison within the sanctuary, their voices resonated with gratitude and praise, filling the hallowed space with the music of worship. They sang with their souls aflame with reverence.

In Hebrew, there are two words for "bless": *esher* and *barak*. When God blesses, it is His gracious action, not ours, and whether people deserve this favor is often irrelevant. *Esher* signifies a state of bliss resulting from human actions, while *barak* implies God granting unmerited blessings, and in another context, it can mean bowing down, kneeling, or worshipping. When humans say they bless God, it is an appeal for God to treat us with grace and kindness, focusing on His favor rather than material blessings.[2] In Psalm 134:1–2, the Levites *barak* God, bowing down, worshipping Him, and asking for His grace as they faithfully serve Him throughout the night. In 134:3, they praise Him as the Creator of heaven and earth and the source of all blessings. Zion symbolizes the presence of God, as His Temple was located in the city of Zion at the time.

---

1 The Babylonian Talmud, Seder Kodashim, Menachot (https://www.sefaria.org/Menachot), 110a, 8.

2 Bertril A. Baird, *The Admiral Gift, Vol 1: Today's First-Century Apostle* (Eugene, OR: Wipf & Stock, 2010), 133–134.

The ABC (Abstract to Brick Concrete)

Bless—General Definition:[3]

- To hallow or consecrate by religious rite, word, or the sign of the cross; to invoke divine care; praise.

Bless—Biblical Definition:

- To bestow a temporal spiritual or earthly gift (how God blesses us); To worship and thank God for His mercies (how we bless God).

The FAST (Focused, Actionable Steps to Take)

Be a channel of God's favor, grace, and kindness to those around you through acts of kindness, encouraging words, heartfelt prayers, and generous giving.

Example: In his daily life, Jordan acts as a conduit for God's favor and kindness, offering prayers for family, friends, and those in need. He extends this prayerful care to others facing difficulties and consistently shares words of encouragement, hope, and kindness in his conversations, recognizing their profound impact on people's emotions and perspectives. Through these actions, Jordan embodies the role of being a vessel for God's love and compassion in the lives of those he interacts with.

---

3 "Bless," Merriam-Webster.com, accessed October 23, 2023, https://www.merriam-webster.com.

25

The Kingdom United—Unity, Love, Peace

*Look, how good and how pleasant it is when **brothers dwell together in unity**. It is **like the fragrant oil upon the head, running down upon the beard, the beard of Aaron, that runs down upon the edges of his robes**. It is **like the dew of Hermon that runs down upon the mountains of Zion, because there Yahweh commanded the blessing—life forever**.*

Psalm 133:1–3

So all the tribes of Israel came to David at Hebron, and they said, "Here we are, we are your flesh and blood."

Second Samuel 5:1

PSALM 133 WAS written by King David when the kingdom of Israel united under his leadership.[1] The second verse, with its imagery of fragrant oil flowing from Aaron's head to the skirts of his garment, symbolizes both the joy of

---

1 John Calvin, *John Calvin's Bible Commentaries on the Psalms 119 - 150* (Loschberg, Germany: Jazzybee Verlag, 2017), 110–111.

unity and the divine mission for the kingdom of Israel. The high priest, Aaron, acted as the intermediary between God and Israel. Similarly, the Israelites were chosen to serve as intermediaries between God and all nations, essentially taking on the role of priests for the world. Through this mission, they were to become the conduit for the abundant blessings to flow to the rest of the world.

In Psalm 133:3, the psalmist beautifully illustrates their brotherly love and unity with the imagery of the dew of Hermon. Mount Hermon, the loftiest peak in Israel, is known for its life-sustaining dew, which descends upon the mountains of Zion. The dew of Hermon provides moisture to its arid surroundings. David conveys that God's blessing, which includes unity, love, and peace, is comparable to the refreshing dew of Hermon. It not only fills the kingdom of Israel but also overflows, extending its reach to other nations.

> Therefore I, the prisoner in the Lord, exhort you to live in a manner worthy of the calling with which you were called: with all humility and gentleness, with patience, putting up with one another in love, being eager to keep the unity of the Spirit in the bond of peace; one body and one Spirit (just as also you were called with one hope of your calling), one Lord, one faith, one baptism, one God and Father of all, who *is* over all, and through all, and in all. (Eph. 4:1–6)
>
> To all these *things add* love, which is *the* bond of perfection. (Col. 3:14)

Apostle Paul emphasizes that love, firmly rooted in Christ, serves as the unifying force that binds together all virtues and individuals, transcending differences and bringing followers of Christ together in a shared purpose of serving Him. This unity in harmony characterizes the community of Christ's dedicated followers, illustrating the power of love to bridge gaps and create a sense of oneness among them.

The practice of servanthood further strengthens unity by fostering a spirit of selfless service and humility. When individuals within the community adopt a servanthood mindset, they willingly put the needs of others above their own, much like Christ, who exemplified this by washing the feet of His disciples (John 13:4–5, 12–17). This selfless dedication deepens their connection and becomes a powerful catalyst for unity among Christians.

> The one who does not love does not know God, because God is love. (1 John 4:8)

Love lies at the very core of God's essence. Love acts as a binding force, uniting people wherever it prevails. This understanding establishes unity as a manifestation of God's presence among humanity.

The ABC (Abstract to Brick Concrete)

Unity—General Definition:[2]

- The quality or state of not being multiple; a condition of harmony; the quality or state of being made one.

Unity—Biblical Definition:

- Oneness in harmony, driven by the shared purpose of serving Christ.

The FAST (Focused, Actionable Steps to Take)

Practice humility and servanthood toward fellow Christians. By doing so, you create an atmosphere of mutual support and selflessness that contributes to achieving and sustaining unity within your faith community.

---

[2] "Unity," Merriam-Webster.com, accessed October 23, 2023, https://www.merriam-webster.com.

Example 1: Henry and Elijah run a cooking ministry in their church, focused on preparing and delivering meals to fellow members during times of need, such as illness, accidents, loss, or financial crisis. Their cooking ministry demonstrates servanthood and unity within their church community, offering support, nourishment, and care when it is needed most. Their efforts reflect the love and compassion that bind their faith community together.

Example 2: Fernando assists non-native speakers during church services and events by providing language translation, both from English to Spanish and vice versa. He stands by their side, translating prayers, sermons, and messages, ensuring that everyone can actively participate and feel connected. His commitment fosters unity among diverse members of the church.

Example 3: Sophia assists elderly church members in accessing online resources, teaching them to use devices and access church websites and social media. She fosters connections among them through virtual gatherings, ensuring their active participation in online church resources.

26

Vanity of Vanities—
The Preacher and Paul

*Remember your Creator in the days of your youth—
before the days of trouble come and the years draw near
when you will say, "I find no pleasure in them!" Before
the sun, the light, the moon, and the stars darken and the
clouds return after the rain. When the guards of the house
tremble, and the men of strength are bent; the grinders
cease because they are few, and those looking through the
windows see dimly. When the doors on the street are shut,
when the sound of the grinding mill is low; one rises up
to the sound of the bird, and all the daughters of song are
brought low. They are afraid of heights, and terrors are on
the road. The almond tree blossoms, and the grasshopper
draws itself along, and desire fails because man goes to his
eternal home, and the mourners go about in the streets.
Before the silver cord is snapped and the golden bowl is
broken; and the jar at the foundation is broken, and the
wheel at the cistern is broken. The dust returns to the earth
as it was, and the breath returns to God who gave it.*

Ecclesiastes 12:1–7

THE PREACHER conveys a clear message to the young: remember that God personally created each of you, breathing life into your souls. Understand that mortal life is fleeting, and death is inevitable. You will be held accountable for both your good and bad deeds in the divine judgment. Turn to Him during your prime, nurturing your faith, hope, and love while your faculties are at their peak rather than in the frailty of old age.

"The sun and the light, and the moon and the stars are darkened" refers to a person's loss of power, standing, position, and authority as one ages and loses the abilities they once had. "The clouds return after the rain" means one calamity after another overwhelms the elderly person, who is already in a weakened state. The preacher uses metaphors to represent the challenges of advanced age: hair going gray and getting thinner, declining eyesight and hearing, weakened teeth and bones, disrupted sleep, and diminishing passion and desires.

The preacher then redirects his attention to the process of dying, which encompasses the cessation of the brain ("golden bowl"), the spinal cord ("silver cord"), the lungs ("jar at the foundation"), and the wheel at the cistern ("heart"). He also describes what happens to the person upon death: their body decomposes into dust, and their soul returns to their creator.

> "Vanity of vanities!" says the Teacher. "Everything *is* vanity!" (Eccles. 12:8)

> For I decided not to know anything among you except Jesus Christ and him crucified. (1 Cor. 2:2)

> *More than that, I* even consider all *things* to be loss because of the surpassing greatness of the knowledge of Christ Jesus my Lord, for the sake of whom I have suffered the loss of all *things*, and consider *them* dung, in order that I may gain Christ. (Phil. 3:8)

In Ecclesiastes 12:8, the word "vanity" is the Hebrew term *hebel*, which can be translated as "vapor," "vain," "absurd," or "meaningless" in English.[1] The meaning of this word *hebel* is amplified by its threefold repetition in this verse. The preacher previously clarified that when he proclaims "vanity," he is referring to things under the sun, thus excluding God and His grace (Eccles. 1:2–3). Thus, he declared that all earthly matter is absolutely vain, absurd, or meaningless. Interestingly, the apostle Paul echoes this message in the New Testament. In First Corinthians 2:2, Paul declares he decided not to know anything other than Christ and His crucifixion. In Philippians 3:8, he expresses the utter vanity of the secular world by revealing he considers secular matters as dung due to the surpassing greatness of the knowledge of Christ.

The similarity between the preacher and the apostle Paul lies in their profound understanding of the transient nature of worldly pursuits when contrasted with the enduring value of spiritual wisdom and the knowledge of God.

The wise preacher explored the futility of worldly endeavors in the book of Ecclesiastes. He described the emptiness and meaninglessness of human achievements, emphasizing that all the riches, power, and pleasures of the world ultimately fail to bring lasting fulfillment. The preacher realized that a life solely dedicated to the pursuit of worldly gain leads to disappointment and disillusionment. He recognized that true wisdom comes from recognizing the temporal nature of earthly pursuits and turning one's focus toward God and His divine revelations.

The apostle Paul arrived at a similar conclusion in the New Testament. He was a man of great learning, a former Pharisee who had ardently pursued knowledge and religious devotion. However, after his conversion to Christianity, Paul had a profound transformation. He declared that he counted all his previous achievements as loss and considered them worthless

---

1 George R. Knight, *Exploring Ecclesiastes and Song of Solomon: A Devotional Commentary* (Hagerstown, MD: Review and Herald, 2006), 34–37.

compared to the surpassing greatness of knowing Christ. In his letters, Paul emphasized the significance of spiritual wisdom and the knowledge of God through Christ, prioritizing the eternal over the transient.

In essence, both the preacher and Paul recognized that the pursuit of earthly wealth, knowledge, and pleasures, while not inherently evil, could lead to a sense of emptiness and disappointment when detached from a deeper understanding of God and His divine wisdom. They both emphasize the ultimate value of focusing on God and the spiritual realm, as this is where true meaning and fulfillment can be found. Their shared insight echoes throughout the Bible, offering profound wisdom for those seeking a deeper understanding of the meaning of life.

The ABC (Abstract to Brick Concrete)

Vanity—General Definition:[2]

- An inflated pride in oneself; something that is vain, empty, or valueless.

Vanity—Biblical Definition:

- The pursuit of worldly success, wealth, and pleasure—which is empty and meaningless, since the only true fulfillment is found in a deeper relationship with God.

The FAST (Focused, Actionable Steps to Take)

Redirect your attention away from the temporary and shallow aspects of worldly success. Instead, center your focus on cultivating an enduring and purposeful relationship with God while serving fellow Christians. Regularly evaluate your actions and priorities to confirm their alignment with this perspective.

---

2 "Vanity," Merriam-Webster.com, accessed October 23, 2023, https://www.merriam-webster.com.

Example: Every morning, Oliver starts his day with a moment of reflection. He takes a few minutes for prayer or meditation, centering his focus on God and eternal values. He sets daily Bible verses and spiritual quotes as wallpapers on his phone and computer. These reminders help him keep his priorities aligned with what truly matters in his daily life, serving as a constant reinforcement, emphasizing the transient and shallow nature of worldly pursuits. He relies on the enduring truths in the teachings of Christ to guide his actions and decisions throughout the day, staying focused on what truly matters in the face of vanity.

27

The Sovereign Ruler—Yahweh

Yahweh is king; he clothes himself with majesty. Yahweh clothes himself; he girds himself with might. Yes, **the** *world is established* **so that** *it will not be moved. Your throne is established from of old; you* **are** *from everlasting.* **The** *rivers have lifted up, O Yahweh;* **the** *rivers have lifted up their* **rumbling;** *the rivers have lifted up their pounding.* **Mightier** *than the rumblings of many waters,* **mightier than** *the* **mighty** *breakers of* **the** *sea, Yahweh on high* **is** *mighty. Your testimonies are fully reliable. Holiness is fitting for your house, O Yahweh,* **forever.**

Psalm 93:1–5

PSALM 93 IS A powerful hymn exalting Yahweh's sovereignty over all creation. It portrays Him as a reigning King, adorned with divine authority, dignity, and glory. The world will not be moved because His eternal kingship would remain unshaken by any opposition. He has ruled from ancient times, continues to reign today, and will extend His rule into the future. God's established order will not falter, unaffected by human sin, natural forces, or the passage of time. Everything aligns with His eternal designs, and His will prevails.

Psalm 93:3 describes the enemies as rising like the roaring waves of the sea, tumultuous and fierce. However, their clamor transforms into the sound of these waves breaking into foam at the presence of Yahweh and His people. Even amid the storm, Yahweh's supremacy remains unshaken. The most formidable threats to His heavenly kingdom are like waves crashing and dissolving at His feet.

In 93:5, the psalmist extols the faithfulness of Yahweh's redeeming word, delivering His chosen people from their adversaries. The Scriptures consistently depict Yahweh's law as flawless, life-sustaining, eternal, holy, and righteous (Ps. 19:7–8; 33:4; 119:137–138, 172; Isa. 40:8; Rom. 7:12). Christ highlighted three essential elements of this law: mercy, justice, and faithfulness (Matt. 23:23). He exercises His sovereign rule over all nations with His perfect decrees, a testament to His divine majesty. He does not tolerate evil and eternally upholds justice in His presence. His "house" is the heavenly Temple filled with His holiness, as exclaimed by the prophet Isaiah (Isa. 6:1–3).

Holiness signifies God's transcendence beyond the limitations of space and time. He exists outside the natural world as the supernatural and wholly distinct One. While God interacts with the world, His holiness sets Him apart, distinguishing Him from the created order.[1] This holiness unequivocally separates Him from everything else. Holiness signifies God's separation from the world, while His immanence signifies His intimate presence and interaction within it.[2] The psalmist is expressing the idea that the place dedicated to God should be set apart from worldly impurities

---

1 Emil Brunner, *The Christian Doctrine of God: Dogmatics: Volume I* (Eugene, OR: Wipf and Stock, 2014), 158.

2 Naomi Koltun-Fromm, *Hermeneutics of Holiness: Ancient Jewish and Christian Notions of Sexuality and Religious Community* (Oxford: Oxford University Press, 2010), 63–67.

and wholly devoted to the sacred, mirroring His divine sanctity, righteousness, and glory.

> Or do you not know that your body is the temple of the Holy Spirit *who is* in you, whom you have from God, and you are not your own? (1 Cor. 6:19)

> And what agreement *does the* temple of God *have* with idols? For we are the temple of the living God, just as God said,
>> "I will live in them and will walk about *among them*, and I will be their God and they will be my people." (2 Cor. 6:16)

Through His precious blood, believers in Christ receive transformative purification. The Holy Spirit graciously takes up residence within those who have been cleansed by Christ, making every Christian a vessel for God's Spirit and thus, His sacred Temple. With this divine dwelling comes a sacred calling: to manifest God's holiness in their daily lives. To mirror His holiness, believers must lead lives set apart from the secular world around them. This distinct way of living places a central emphasis on the practice of love, extending not only to love for God but also love for fellow Christians. It also involves exercise of faith by following His law and living according to His teachings. To sustain this way of living, they must firmly anchor their hope in Christ's eternal kingdom, rising above the transient aspects of this earthly existence.

The ABC (Abstract to Brick Concrete)

Sovereignty—General Definition:[3]

- Supreme power; freedom from external control; controlling influence; supreme excellence.

---

[3] "Sovereignty," Merriam-Webster.com, accessed October 23, 2023, https://www.merriam-webster.com.

Sovereignty—Biblical Definition:
- The supreme and absolute authority of God over all creation, reflecting His unrivaled rulership and dominion

The FAST (Focused, Actionable Steps to Take)

Acknowledging God's sovereignty, strive to fulfill your daily responsibilities with unwavering diligence and integrity. Recognize that God has purposefully positioned you in specific roles, and by performing these tasks with excellence, you play a part in His greater plan for your life and the world.

Example 1: As a businesswoman, Amelia fully acknowledges God's sovereignty in her business practice. She works with integrity and diligence, seeing it as part of God's plan. Her business decisions align with her Christian values, reflecting her faith and commitment to making a positive impact.

Example 2: In his role as an educator, Alex embraces the concept of God's sovereignty. He sees teaching as a part of God's plan for him and his students. His teaching methods and interactions with students are guided by Christian values, emphasizing respect, compassion, and the nurturing of their potential.

Example 3: Nathalie, as a grocery store cashier, doesn't view her job merely as a means of earning a living but as a part of God's purpose for her life at this point in time. In every transaction, each interaction with customers, and her friendly demeanor, she embodies Christian values of kindness, patience, and service. Her dedication to providing excellent customer service and bringing a smile to people's faces is a direct expression of her faith.

28

A Man Spared by Divine Providence—Baruch

I [Jeremiah] bought the field from Hanamel, the son of my uncle, that was *at Anathoth. I weighed out to him the money, seventeen silver shekels. And I signed on the letter and sealed* it, *and I called witnesses as witness, and I weighed out the money on a set of scales. Then I took the deed of the purchase, the sealed* copy containing *the commandments and the rules, together with the* one *that was open. And I gave the deed of the purchase to Baruch the son of Neriah, the son of Mahseiah, in the presence of Hanamel,* the son of *my uncle, and* in the presence of *the witnesses who signed the deed of the purchase,* in the presence of *the Judeans who were sitting in the courtyard of the guard. And I commanded Baruch* in their presence, saying, *'Thus says Yahweh of hosts, the God of Israel, "Take these deeds, this deed of the purchase, the sealed one, and this opened deed, and you must put them in an* earthenware jar *so that they may be kept preserved many days." For thus says Yahweh of hosts, the God of Israel: "Houses and fields and vineyards will again be bought in this land."'*

Jeremiah 32:9–15

IN THE BOOK OF Jeremiah, we encounter Baruch, the fearless scribe who wrote down Jeremiah's prophecies of judgment and condemnation upon all nations, even at the peril of his own life. The name "Baruch" is an English variation of *Berechiah*, originating from the Hebrew term *Baruk*, which signifies a divine, unconditional blessing.[1] Before dedicating himself to the ministry, his professional work as a scribe is depicted in Jeremiah 32, where Jeremiah purchases land from his cousin Hanamel at Anathoth. This purchase was a bold prophetic declaration that God would indeed gather and restore the remnant of Israel to their homeland.

A name featuring the addition of a paternal ancestor's name is called a patronym. A double patronym is the addition of the father's and grandfather's name after a person's given name. In ancient Israel, the use of a double patronym was a distinguishing mark of royal and noble families.[2] In 32:12, Baruch's name bears a double patronym, signifying his heritage from a distinguished family. Just as with other professions of that era, the role of a scribe passed down through generations.[3]

Seriah, Baruch's brother, is mentioned in Jeremiah 51 as a high officer in the service of King Zedekiah. He carries out various scribal duties, including the task of reading a scroll aloud (51:59–64).

Furthermore, his paternal grandfather, Maaseiah, served King Joisah as the commander of Jerusalem and repaired the holy Temple in the 18th year of his reign (2 Chron. 34:8). The

---

1 J. Edward Wright, *Baruch Ben Neriah: From Biblical Scribe to Apocalyptic Seer* (Columbia, SC: University of South Carolina Press, 2003), 1.

2 James Muilenburg, "Baruch the Scribe," in *Proclamation and Presence* (Richmond, VA: John Knox, 1970), 23.

3 Jack R. Lundbom, "Baruch, Seraiah, and Expanded Colophons in the Book of Jeremiah," *The Journal for the Study of the Old Testament*, Vol. 11, Issue 36, 1986, 89–114.

historical account of his family members serving kings over multiple generations also supports the notion that Baruch likely held the position of a royal scribe before his divine calling. In 1977, a significant archaeological discovery came to light, providing compelling evidence for their heritage. Among the findings was a seal impression in a royal archive inscribed with "Belonging to Berechiah [Baruch], [the son of] Neriah, the scribe."[4] Moreover, they uncovered the original seal, bearing the inscription "Belonging to Seraiah, [the son of] Neriah."[5] This discovery essentially confirmed his lineage as a royal scribe.

> In the fourth year of Jehoiakim the son of Josiah, the king of Judah, this word came to Jeremiah from Yahweh, *saying*, "Take for yourself *a scroll* and you must write on it all the words that I have spoken to you against Israel, and against Judah, and against all the nations, from *the* day *that* I spoke to you, from the days of Josiah, and until this day. Perhaps *when* the house of Judah hears all the disasters that I *am* planning to do to them, then they may turn back each one from his evil way, and I will forgive their guilt and their sin." (Jer. 36:1–3)

Yahweh called Jeremiah to prophesy in the thirteenth year of Josiah's thirty-one-year reign (25:3). Fast forward to the fourth year of Jehoiakim, Josiah's son and successor, and we find ourselves in Jeremiah's twenty-third year as a prophet. This period is pivotal in the kingdom of Judah, as it unfolds eighteen years before the destruction of Jerusalem. God instructs Jeremiah to put His words in writing, expanding the audience from the local Jerusalem population to encompass people across nations and generations. The written prophecies are not merely a record of

---

4 Nahman Avigad, "Baruch the Scribe and Jerahmeel the King's Son," *Israel Exploration Journal*, Vol. 28, No. 1/2, 1978, 52–56.

5 Nahman Avigad, "The Seal of Seraiah (Son of) Neriah," *H.L. Ginsberg Volume* , Eretz Israel 14 (Jerusalem, Israel: Israel Exploration Society, 1978), 86–87, 125.

history; they also offer timeless lessons and insights that apply to the present and future generations. They serve as a living testament to the fulfillment of God's word throughout history and provide valuable guidance and wisdom for those living today. The written word of God also offered King Jehoiakim and his council a distinct advantage. It allowed for careful, repeated reading and contemplation, promoting a deeper understanding of His message. In His boundless mercy God aimed to open the door for their spiritual conversion and the potential forgiveness of their transgressions. Even in the midst of His wrath, God extended His grace, mercy, and compassion by repetitively sending messages to warn them.

> Then Jeremiah called Baruch the son of Neriah, and Baruch wrote from the mouth of Jeremiah all the words of Yahweh that he had spoken to him on *a scroll.* Jeremiah instructed Baruch, *saying,* "I *am* held back, I am not able to enter the temple of Yahweh. So you must go and you shall read aloud from the scroll that you have written from my mouth the words of Yahweh in the hearing of the people *in* the temple of Yahweh on a day of fast, and also you shall read aloud in the hearing of all those of Judah who came from their towns. Perhaps their plea will fall *before* Yahweh and each one will turn away from his evil way, for great *is* the anger and wrath that Yahweh pronounced against these people." Baruch the son of Neriah did all that Jeremiah the prophet instructed him, to read aloud from the scroll the words of Yahweh *in* the temple of Yahweh. (Jer. 36:4–8)

Jeremiah enlisted the aid of his scribe, Baruch, to assist in fulfilling his divine mission. Baruch meticulously transcribed God's message as spoken by the prophet Jeremiah. The process commenced during the fourth year of Jehoiakim's reign, with the scroll being publicly read in the fifth year, during the ninth month. Considering this timeline, the writing of the scroll may have taken as long as a year or more to complete.

Shockingly, once the scroll was complete, Jeremiah was unable to enter the holy Temple. It seems that he was somehow disqualified or prevented from entering the holy Temple, yet the cause for this restriction, whether due to physical ailment, ceremonial impurity, royal or priestly prohibition, or divine command, remains unknown. While there are some theories that Jeremiah may have been confined to a prison cell, there is no record of his imprisonment during Jehoiakim's reign.[6] Additionally, in Jeremiah 36:26, both Jeremiah and Baruch hide from Jehoiakim when he sends his men to apprehend them. If Jeremiah had already been imprisoned, he would not have had to go into hiding to avoid arrest.

Jeremiah then entrusted Baruch with the responsibility of reading the completed scroll to the people at the holy Temple. He specifically chose a fast day in the ninth month when the largest crowds gathered, including people from various areas of Judah. This wasn't a common annual fast but a robust national response to a specific issue, perhaps related to famine, infectious disease, or the growing threat posed by the Babylonians.[7] Unfortunately, the currently available historical records do not provide a clear explanation for the cause of this national reaction. However, it presented the prime opportunity for God's message to be proclaimed to the Jews gathered from all areas of the nation. Jeremiah hoped that this act would encourage them to supplicate to Yahweh, potentially averting the impending doom of the nation.

> In the fifth year of Jehoiakim, the son of Josiah, the king of Judah, in the ninth month, all the people in Jerusalem and all the people who came from the towns of Judah to Jerusalem

---

6 Jean Calvin, *Commentaries on the Book of the Prophet Jeremiah and the Lamentations* (Edinburgh, Scotland: Calvin Translation Society, 1854), 329–331.

7 John Gill, *An Exposition of the Old Testament* (London: Mathews and Leigh, 1810), 606–607.

proclaimed a fast *before* Yahweh. Then Baruch read aloud from the scroll the words of Jeremiah *in* the temple of Yahweh, in the chamber of Gemariah, the son of Shaphan, the secretary, in the upper courtyard *at* the entrance of the New Gate of the temple of Yahweh in the hearing of all the people.

When Micaiah, the son of Gemariah, the son of Shaphan, heard all the words of Yahweh from the scroll, he went down *to* the house of the king, to the chamber of the secretary, and look, all the officials *were* sitting there: Elishama the secretary, and Delaiah, the son of Shemaiah, and Elnathan, the son of Achbor, and Gemariah, the son of Shaphan, and Zedekiah, the son of Hananiah, and all the *other* officials. And Micaiah told them all the words that he had heard at the reading aloud of Baruch from the scroll in the hearing of the people.

Then all the officials sent Jehudi, the son of Nethaniah, the son of Shelemiah, the son of Cushi, to Baruch, *saying*, "The scroll that you read aloud from in the hearing of the people, take it in your hand and come." And Baruch the son of Neriah took the scroll in his hand and he came to them. (Jer. 36:9–14)

Baruch cleverly selected the chamber of the scribe Gemariah for the scroll reading at the holy Temple. He was one of the few faithful servants of Yahweh remaining in the kingdom of Judah. Baruch likely knew Gemariah from his past service as a royal scribe in Jerusalem. Gemariah's brother, Ahikam, and his father, Shaphan, played pivotal roles in the religious revival of King Josiah (39:14; 2 Chron. 34:18–21). Moreover, Ahikam had previously come to Jeremiah's aid when the prophet was in great danger (Jer. 26:24). Given the insight and foreknowledge Baruch possessed, his choice of location was undoubtedly strategic.

Baruch proclaimed the divine message of condemnation and judgment and God's call for repentance to the multitudes gathered at the holy Temple on a fast day. Micaiah, son of Gemariah, heard Baruch's message and promptly rushed to the chamber of

Elishama, where he found Gemariah, the royal secretary Elishama, and several other elders and nobles. Upon hearing what transpired, Elishama urgently sent his subordinate to bring Baruch into his chamber. As Baruch entered the room, a palpable tension gripped the air, like the calm before a storm. Baruch clutched the sacred scroll, brimming with messages of divine judgment and condemnation. In that moment, the eyes of the esteemed officials in the kingdom of Judah were fixed on him, their collective anticipation throbbing in the air like a tightly wound spring.

> They said to him, "Sit please and read it aloud in our hearing." So Baruch read aloud in their hearing. *And then*, the moment of their hearing all the words, *they turned to one another in alarm* and they said to Baruch, "We must certainly report all these words to the king!" Then they asked Baruch, *saying*, "Tell us please, how did you write all these words, from his mouth?" And Baruch said to them, "From his mouth. He dictated to me all these words and I *was* writing on the scroll with the ink." Then the officials said to Baruch, "Go, hide yourself, you and Jeremiah, and let not a man know where you *are*." (Jer. 36:15–19)

Baruch, undeterred and resolute, conveyed the entire word of God. The officials listened intently as every word struck them with sheer terror. The officers, their voices trembling with anxiety, sought assurance from Baruch regarding the message's authenticity. He confirmed that every word inscribed upon the scroll came directly from the prophet Jeremiah. Elishama and his council then decided to deliver the message to King Jehoiakim. Fully aware of King Jehoiakim's tyrannical temper, they urged Baruch to take Jeremiah with him and find a place to hide.

> They went to the king, *to the* courtyard, and they *put* the scroll for safe-keeping in the chamber of Elishama the secretary, and they reported all the words in the hearing of the king. Then the king sent Jehudi to take the scroll, and he took it from the chamber of Elishama the secretary, and Jehudi read it aloud in

the hearing of the king, and in the hearing of all the officials who stood next to the king. Now the king *was* sitting *in* the quarters of the winter in the ninth month, and a fire-pot *was* burning *before* him. *And then,* as Jehudi read three or four columns, he would cut it up in pieces with the knife of the scribe, and he would throw *it* into the fire that *was* in the fire-pot until the whole of the scroll *was* consumed in the fire that was in the fire-pot. And the king and any of his servants who heard all these words were not startled, and they did not tear their garments. And even *when* Elnathan, Delaiah, and Gemariah urged the king not to burn the scroll, he would not listen to them. And the king commanded Jerahmeel, the son of the king, and Seraiah, the son of Azriel, and Shelemiah, the son of Abdeel, to arrest Baruch the secretary and Jeremiah the prophet, but Yahweh hid them. (Jer. 36:20–26)

Elishama and his council had stashed Baruch's scroll in his chamber, attempting to protect it from King Jehoiakim. Nevertheless, when the king received notice of the prophetic messages, he instantly ordered his subordinate to retrieve and recite the contents of the scroll. Unfortunately, their efforts to safeguard it proved futile under the grip of this tyrannical ruler. Struck by the word of God, Jehoiakim felt immense guilt and shame, which fueled his vehement rejection of it.

In his winter residence, King Jehoiakim had a pot of coals burning beside his throne. As the reading progressed, every three to four lines met the sharp blade of the king's penknife, and those segments were cast into the fire. This procedure continued until the entire scroll had been reduced to ashes in the searing flames. This destruction was not a rash act but a deliberate and calculated affront to Yahweh. Three courageous individuals, Gemariah, Elnathan, and Delaiah, stepped forward to make an intercession, urging the king not to burn the scroll. However, their efforts proved futile. The king, undeterred, took it a step further, dispatching a unit to apprehend the prophet Jeremiah and his scribe

Baruch. Protected by divine intervention, Jeremiah and Baruch successfully evaded the king's envoys and remained unharmed.

> The word of Yahweh came to Jeremiah after the king burned the scroll and the words that Baruch wrote from the mouth of Jeremiah, *saying*, "*Take again* for yourself another scroll and write on it all the former words that were in the first scroll which Jehoiakim, the king of Judah, has burned. And concerning Jehoiakim, the king of Judah, you shall say, 'Thus says Yahweh, "You have burned this scroll, *saying*, 'Why have you written in it, *saying*, "The king of Babylon will certainly come and he will destroy this land, and he will cause to disappear from it humankind and animals"?'" *Therefore* thus says Yahweh concerning Jehoiakim, the king of Judah, "There will not be for him *one who* sits on the throne of David. His dead body will be thrown out to the heat in the day and to the frost in the night. I will punish him, and his offspring, and his servants for their guilt, and I will bring on them, and on the inhabitants of Jerusalem, and on the people of Judah all the disaster with which I have threatened them, but they would not listen."'" Then Jeremiah took another scroll and gave it to Baruch the son of Neriah, the secretary, and he wrote on it from the mouth of Jeremiah all the words of the scroll that Jehoiakim, the king of Judah, had burned in the fire, and furthermore was added to them many words like these. (Jer. 36:27–32)

In his place of concealment, Jeremiah received a divine command to rewrite the scroll King Jehoiakim had destroyed. The revised scroll contained four specific threats directed toward him: First, he would have no descendant to firmly occupy David's throne. Second, Jeremiah predicted a violent and dishonorable death for Jehoiakim, emphasizing the indignity of being left unburied. Thirdly, God's punishment would extend to the king's family and servants, ensuring they would share in the retribution. Fourth and lastly, the people of Judah and Jerusalem would experience the calamity foretold by Yahweh's prophets for years.

The word that Jeremiah the prophet spoke to Baruch, the son of Neriah, at his writing these words on a scroll from the mouth of Jeremiah, in the fourth year of Jehoiakim, the son of Josiah, the king of Judah, *saying*, "Thus says Yahweh, the God of Israel, to you, O Baruch: 'You said, "Woe please to me, for Yahweh has added sorrow to my pain. I am weary in my groaning and I do not find rest."' Thus you will say to him: Thus says Yahweh, "Look, what I have built I *am* about to tear down, and what I have planted I *am* about to pluck up, it *is* all the land. And you, *do* you seek great *things* for yourself? Do not seek *great things*, for look, I *am* about to bring disaster upon all flesh," *declares* Yahweh, "but to you I will give your life as booty in all the places where you may go."'" (Jer. 45:1–5)

These interactions described in this passage took place in the fourth year of Jehoiakim, before Baruch proclaimed the word of God at the holy Temple. Thus, this passage should be understood in the context of Jeremiah chapter 36. Baruch mourning over his life being at risk indicates that this event likely took place while Jeremiah and Baruch were in hiding from King Jehoiakim.

The heartwrenching lamentation of Baruch in 45:3 captures his agony with the following words: woe, sorrow, pain, groaning, weariness, and restlessness. In the same verse, he uses a personal pronoun five times: me, my, I, my, and I. Baruch, born into a highly educated royal scribe family, bore the weight of society's and his family's expectations for a great career and lasting legacy. During this period, serving as a prominent Prophet's scribe held great prestige and honor. However, their ministry began to falter, and they were falsely accused of treason against the country. They found themselves in a hidden place, pursued by King Jehoiakim with this deeply dishonorable accusation. Amid this daunting turn of events, Baruch was also devastated by the crushing failure of his own lofty ambitions. He believed he was falling short of the expectations he, his family, and society had for him. This situation is comparable to the son of a U.S. government secretary being pursued for arrest on charges of collaborating with a foreign power like Russia, not only tarnishing his reputation but also shattering the hopes of his prestigious family.

Yahweh met his secular desires with compassion and grace instead of wrath and fury. God kindly reasoned with Baruch, gently guiding him to realign his perspective. He revealed to Baruch the futility of his pursuit of honor, prestige, and power in the kingdom of Judah. These riches and influences were, like sandcastles on the shore, soon to disappear with the impending destruction of Judah. Just as the tide washes away transient accomplishments, the end of his country would eclipse these fleeting ambitions. Instead, God promised Baruch that He would spare his life through all the trials in the process, and that after the fall of Judah, He would provide him with a lasting and precious gift amid the tumultuous times.

Baruch aspired to establish a legacy as a scribe in the kingdom of Judah, but God had him transcribe the book of Jeremiah instead. This book later found its place in the Bible, its words reaching every corner of the globe and spanning countless generations for over two millennia. This achievement far exceeded his initial aspirations in ways he could never have fathomed.

The New Testament delves deeper into the topic of personal ambition, categorizing it into two types. Baruch's initial ambition aligns with what the apostles James and Paul referred to as "selfish ambition." They describe it as an earthly, unspiritual, impure, and even demonic force that disrupts the unity among believers. They caution against ambitions of this kind, which can prompt evil actions (James 3:14–16; Phil. 2:3–4; Rom. 2:8–9; 2 Cor. 12:20–21). Paul is clear that selfish ambition can also lead to disqualification from inheriting the kingdom of heaven (Gal. 5:19–21). "Holy ambition" refers to an unyielding desire to excel in fulfilling God's mission. This force of unity brings believers together through their shared goal of carrying out God's will (Rom. 15:20–21; 2 Cor. 5:9–10).

The ABC (Abstract to Brick Concrete)

Ambition—General Definition:[8]

- Ambition: An ardent desire for rank, fame, or power; desire to achieve a particular end.

Ambition—Biblical Definition:

- *Selfish Ambition:* An earthly, unspiritual, impure, and even demonic desire for success that incites evil actions and disrupts the unity among believers.
- *Holy Ambition:* An unyielding desire to excel in fulfilling God's mission. This force of unity brings believers together through their shared goal of carrying out God's will.

The FAST (Focused, Actionable Steps to Take)

1. Practice selflessness by prioritizing the needs and well-being of fellow Christians ahead of your own. This approach fosters a mindset of selflessness, which encourages empathy, cooperation, and a focus on collective well-being.

   Example 1: Liam is a young man who works as a professional baseball player. He practices selflessness by providing compassionate end-of-life care to terminally ill fellow Christians who may not have family members or friends to be with them during their final days. He ensures their comfort and peace by tending to their physical, emotional, and spiritual needs with unwavering dedication and empathy.

---

8 "Ambition," Merriam-Webster.com, accessed October 23, 2023, https://www.merriam-webster.com.

Example 2: Grace, a professional painter, extends her artistic talent and compassion by visiting a Christian orphanage to teach painting to young children. With a heart full of warmth and creativity, she arrives with an array of colorful paints, canvases, and brushes, ready to inspire the young minds. She encourages them to unleash their creativity and express themselves through painting. Her smile and encouragement put the children at ease, making them feel safe and valued.

2. To ignite and fuel your holy ambition, actively engage in God's work, compelling you to make more significant contributions to His mission.

   Example 1: Taylor volunteered to raise funds for a Christian organization's missionary work. This initial involvement deepened her connection to God's mission and kindled a growing desire to excel in fulfilling it. As she continued her efforts, her holy ambition grew, leading her to set new spiritual goals, pray fervently, and share her faith more passionately each day.

   Example 2: Nathan directly supports his church's soup kitchen, preparing nourishing meals for those in need. His service aligns with God's mission, spreading love and compassion. His involvement has ignited his holy ambition to excel in this mission and continually find new ways to serve those in need.

29

Locust Locos:
A Loud Call for Repentance—Joel

The word of Yahweh that came to Joel son of Pethuel. Hear this, O elders, and give ear, all the inhabitants of the land. Has this happened in your days? Or the days of your ancestors? Tell it to your children, and your children to their children, and their children to the following generation. What the cutting locust left, the swarming locust has eaten. What the swarming locust left, the hopping locust has eaten. And what the hopping locust left, the destroying locust has eaten.

Joel 1:1–4

THE PROPHET JOEL served in the kingdom of Judah during a time of catastrophic locust infestation. The absence of any mention of the king of Judah at the time can be attributed to its occurrence during the sixth year of the reign of Queen Mother Athaliah.[1] This chronological context places the book of Joel between the Book of Amos and the Book of Hosea.

---
1 Willem S. Prinsloo, *The Theology of the Book of Joel* (Berlin, Germany: Walter de Gruyter & Co., 1985), 1–10.

The prophecy commences by clearly stating its subject (the Leham English Bible gives it the heading "A Lament Over the Land") and its intended recipients, encompassing the political leaders and all inhabitants of the kingdom of Judah. Joel paints a haunting picture of the kingdom of Judah in the throes of a catastrophic locust infestation. They suffered an unrelenting onslaught of the locusts, commencing with the slow and deliberate chewing of their crops. Then came the swarming, a cloud of locusts blotting out the sun, bringing with it despair. The locusts crawled over every inch of their land, leaving behind an absolute desolation. And finally, they consumed all that remained, leaving nothing but barren earth in their wake. The famine that followed was not just an absence of food but a gnawing, insatiable hunger that gripped the people. The pangs of hunger echoed in every corner of Judah. The financial ruin that ensued added to their misery, reducing the once-prosperous kingdom to a state of destitution. This locust infestation was so harrowing that its memory would haunt the descendants for generations to come.

> Wake up, drunkards, and weep!
> Wail, all drinkers of wine, over the new wine,
>   for it is cut off from your mouth.
> Because a nation has *invaded* my land,
>   strong *and beyond counting*.
> Its teeth *are* the teeth of a lion,
>   and its fangs *are those* of a lioness.
> It has made my vine a desolation,
>   and my fig tree a completely splintered stump.
> It has stripped them bare and thrown *them* down;
>   their branches have turned white.
>
> (Joel 1:5–7)

Because you [drunkards] have said,

> "We have *made* a covenant with death,
>   and we have made an agreement with Sheol.

> *The* overwhelming flood, when it passes through,
>> will not come to us,
>
> for we have made lies our refuge,
> and we have hidden ourselves in falsehood."
>> (Isa. 28:15)

Joel urges the drunkards to wake up to witness the extensive destruction caused by the locusts. The biblical definition of "drunkards" is found in 28:15, describing them as those intoxicated with a false sense of security derived from earthly sources such as political alliances, false doctrines, and pagan idol gods. This figurative language emphasizes their foolishness in trusting deceptive and powerless entities instead of turning to their faithful God.

The locusts, typically weak and insignificant creatures, wouldn't ordinarily pose a threat to a nation. However, as the Jews turned away from God, they lost their strength, sinking into a profound state of weakness. To such an extent that even the locusts began to assert dominance over them, much like powerful lions. These locusts arrived as a formidable force, seizing control of the land. Even amid this disgraceful situation, God reaffirmed His claim on them as His people, maintaining ownership of the land, vines, and fig trees. He sent them Joel to deliver His call for repentance.

> Lament like a virgin girded in a sackcloth
>> for the husband of her youth.
>
> The offering and libation are withheld
>> from the house of Yahweh.
>
> The priests mourn,
>> the ministers of Yahweh.
>
> The field is destroyed;
>> the earth mourns
>
> because *the* grain is destroyed,
>> *the* new wine dries up,
>>> *the* olive oil languishes.
>
> Be ashamed, farmers;
>> Wail, vinedressers,

over *the* wheat and over *the* barley,
    because *the* harvest of the field is ruined.
The vine withers
    and the fig tree droops.
The pomegranate tree, and also the palm tree, the apple tree
    —all the trees of the field—are dried up.
Indeed, joy is dried up
    among the sons of men.
Gird yourselves and lament, O priests!
    Wail, *O* ministers of *the* altar!
Come spend the night in sackcloth,
    O ministers of my God,
because offering and libation
    are withheld from the house of your God.
Solemnize a fast!
    Call an assembly!
Gather *the* elders,
    all *of* the inhabitants of the land
in the house of Yahweh your God,
    and cry out to Yahweh.

(Joel 1:8–14)

Joel urges the people to turn to their faithful God, who will provide help as they belong to Him. Relying on pagan idols, political alliances, or false prophets would be futile because they do not have ownership of Judah. Only the true owner, Creator, and God genuinely cared for them and their land. He proclaims a call for repentance to the kingdom of Judah, imploring the priests to gather for a solemn fast. He pleads with the people to renounce sinful acts, humble themselves before God, and cast their sorrow and pain before Him.

Ah! For the day!
For the day of Yahweh is near.
    It will come like destruction from Shaddai.
Is not food cut *off*

>   before our eyes,
> from the house of our God,
>   joy and gladness?
> The seeds shrivel under their clods;
>   the storehouses are desolate.
> The grain storage places are destroyed
>   because grain has dried out.
> How *the* beasts groan;
>   the herds of cattle wander around
> because there is no pasture for them;
>   *the* flocks of sheep are in distress.
> To you, *O* Yahweh, I cry out,
> because fire has devoured
>   the pastures of the desert,
> and flames burned
>   all the trees of the field.
> Also, the beasts of *the* field
>   long for you,
> because the courses of water
>   are dried up,
> and fire has devoured
>   the pastures of the desert.
>
>   (Joel 1:15–20)

The call for repentance is not solely to seek deliverance from the locust affliction; it is an urgent plea to spare them from further divine wrath. He describes the suffering of plants and animals throughout the land, all crying out to God. Astonishingly, the only ones who have not turned to God even in such an agonizing misery are His chosen people.

The ABC (Abstract to Brick Concrete)

Drunkard—General Definition:[2]
- One who frequently impairs their mental and physical abilities by drinking alcohol.

Drunkard—Biblical Definition:
- One who finds false security in deceptive and powerless entities like political alliances, false doctrines, and pagan idols.

The FAST (Focused, Actionable Steps to Take)

Engage in open and honest conversations about your faith with fellow Christians at the end of every month to avoid placing false security in false sources. This practice will help you stay on the right path and provide an opportunity for guidance and support when needed.

Example: At the end of each month, Batinna and her fellow Christians come together to discuss their faith and spiritual journeys. During one meeting, Batinna shared her ongoing struggle with doubts arising from theological debates she encountered online. The other church members provided guidance, shared relevant Bible verses, and offered encouragement to help Batinna address her uncertainties. These direct and candid monthly discussions strengthen their bond and ensure that they stay on the right spiritual path.

---

[2] "Drunkard," Merriam-Webster.com, accessed October 23, 2023, https://www.merriam-webster.com.

30

Rising Stars of Faith

Stories of Exemplary New Christians —The Thessalonians

Paul and Silvanus and Timothy, to the church of the Thessalonians in God the Father and the Lord Jesus Christ. Grace to you and peace. We give thanks to God always concerning all of you, making mention constantly in our prayers, because we *remember your work of faith and labor of love and steadfastness of hope in our Lord Jesus Christ in the presence of our God and Father.*

First Thessalonians 1:1–3

A vision appeared to Paul during the night: a certain Macedonian man was standing there and imploring him and saying, "Come over to Macedonia and *help us!" When he had seen the vision, we [Paul, Silvanus, Luke, Timothy] wanted at once to go away to Macedonia, concluding that God had called us to proclaim the good news to them.*

Acts 16:9–10

WITH A POPULATION of about 200,000 people, the city of Thessalonica held the distinguished position of being the capital city of Macedonia province.[1] It had the privilege of governing its citizens as a free city, even during the Roman Empire's rule.[2] God presented the apostle Paul with a vision of a man in Macedonia pleading for his arrival to offer help. This divine vision ignited a holy zeal within Paul and his ministry companions to embark on a journey to evangelize the region of Macedonia.

In response to the divine calling, they shared the gospel with the people of Thessalonica. Their ministry over three weeks was remarkably successful, leading to the conversion of many individuals who played a key role in building the Thessalonian church (Acts 17:2–4). Following Paul's departure, Silas and Timothy stayed to support and mentor the newly converted. However, they also had to leave shortly afterwards to help spread the gospel in Athens (17:14–15).

In under a year after leaving Thessalonica, Paul sent Timothy back to check on the community (1 Thess. 3:2–3).[3] Six months later, Timothy returned with an overwhelmingly positive report: the Thessalonian believers stood strong in their faith and love despite challenges (3:6).[4] This prompted Paul to write his first letter to the Thessalonians to further encourage them.

> Knowing, brothers *dearly* loved by God, *that he has chosen you.* (1:4)

---

1 Warren W. Wiersbe, *The Bible Exposition Commentary* (Colorado Springs: David C. Cook, 2003), 156–163.

2 George G. Findlay, *The Epistles to the Thessalonians* (Cambridge, England: The University Press, 1898), 9–12.

3 Abraham J. Malherbe, *The Letters to the Thessalonians: A New Translation with Introduction and Commentary* (New Haven, CT: Yale University Press, 2004), 72.

4 Malherbe, 72.

> And will not God surely *see to it that justice is done* to his chosen ones who cry out to him day and night, and will he delay toward them? (Luke 18:7)

> He will send out his angels with a loud trumpet call, and they will gather his elect together from the four winds, from *one* end of heaven to the *other* end of it. . . . Then the king will say to those on his right, "Come, *you* who are blessed by my Father. Inherit the kingdom prepared for you from the foundation of the world!" . . . And these will depart into eternal punishment, but the righteous into eternal life. (Matt. 24:31; 25:34, 46)

Christ made it known that God had predestined certain individuals for salvation and eternal life before the creation of the world. Paul conveyed to the Thessalonian believers that they are among these chosen people.

> Because our gospel did not come to you with word only, but also with power and with the Holy Spirit and with much certainty, just as you know what sort of *people* we became among you for your sake. You became imitators of us and of the Lord, receiving the word in much affliction, with the joy of the Holy Spirit, so that you became an example to all those who believe in Macedonia and in Achaia, for from you the word of the Lord has sounded forth, not only in Macedonia and Achaia, but in every place your faith toward God has gone out, so that we have no need to say anything. For *they* themselves report about us, what sort of welcome we had with you, and how you turned to God from idols to serve *the* living and true God, and to await his Son from heaven, whom he raised from the dead, Jesus, the one who delivers us from the coming wrath. (1 Thess. 1:5–10)

Paul explains that they had embraced the gospel through the work of the Holy Spirit because God had chosen them as His people. He goes on, sharing that he and his ministry companions sought to imitate Christ, and now the Thessalonian believers were following in their footsteps. They were setting an example for the people in Macedonia and Achaia to follow.

In the book of Colossians, Paul elaborates on what it means to imitate Christ. It involves living a life filled with love, compassion, kindness, humility, gentleness, patience, forgiveness, and gratitude. Furthermore, it means studying and applying Christ's teachings, and using them as a basis for teaching, advising, and encouraging one another (Col. 3:12–17). The Thessalonian believers wholeheartedly embraced the example Paul and his ministry companions had set. Their commitment to living out the teachings of Christ not only impacted their local community but also made a lasting impression wherever they shared the gospel.

The ABC (Abstract to Brick Concrete)

Elect—General Definition:[5]

- Carefully selected; one set apart; chosen by divine favor; voted for a position.

Elect—Biblical Definition:

- One predestined for salvation and eternal life before the creation of the world; chosen by God, called through the work of the Holy Spirit, and justified through Christ

The FAST (Focused, Actionable Steps to Take)

As the elect, we must live in a way that aligns with our divine calling (Eph. 4:1). This involves actively practicing our faith, demonstrating Christ's love to the world, and holding steadfast in our hope in Christ.

---

5 "Elect," Merriam-Webster.com, accessed October 23, 2023, https://www.merriam-webster.com.

Example 1: Finn exercised his faith by engaging in faith-based volunteer work in Africa. He immersed himself in the local culture, serving the community during the day and sharing Christ's love in the evenings. This experience deepened his faith while allowing him to impact the lives of others. Finn further expresses his faith by making monthly financial donations to the same ministry group. His consistent support plays a crucial role in sustaining their ministry, ensuring that the impact of his faith reaches beyond borders and into the lives of those in need.

Example 2: Every day, Grey brings an extra lunch to school for a friend in need. This week, he took his friend to his church, introducing him to the welcoming congregation, who create a sense of belonging and warmth in the community.

Example 3: Gemma is committed to bringing hope to challenging regions by translating English Christian sermons, devotionals, and books into Mandarin. Her dedication extends beyond translation as she engages with local communities, sharing her faith and offering support to those in need. Her work reflects unwavering hope in Christ amid adversity.

31
The Feast of Remnants —Haggai

In the second year of King Darius, in the sixth month, on the first day, the word of Yahweh came through Haggai the prophet to Zerubbabel the son of Shealtiel, governor of Judah, and to Joshua the son of Jehozadak, the high priest, saying . . .

Haggai 1:1

On the day of your joy and in your appointed times, at the beginning of your months, you will blow on the trumpets in addition to your burnt offerings and in addition to the sacrifices of your fellowship offerings. And they will be as a memorial for you before your God; I am Yahweh your God.

Numbers 10:10

THE NAME OF THE prophet Haggai is derived from the Hebrew name *haggay*, which means "my feast" or "festal."[1] This is a fitting name for him, because all the prophecies recorded in the book of Haggai were received on feast days. His first

---

1 Pieter A. Verhoef, *The Books of Haggai and Malachi* (Grand Rapids: Eerdmans, 1987), 3–5.

prophecy came on the first day of the month, a day of celebration as noted in Numbers 10:10. The second and third prophecies occurred on the seventh day of the Tabernacle Feast and on the day the foundation of the second Temple was laid (Hag. 2:1, 18; Lev. 23:34–36). These occurrences highlight the symbolism of feasting, signifying the joyous return from a seven-decade-long exile and the promise of future glory. Haggai was the first prophet to speak to the post-exilic community upon their return from the Babylonian captivity.[2] His first prophecy was directed toward Zerubbabel, the governor of Judah, and Joshua, the high priest.

Following his conquest of the Babylonian Empire, Persian King Cyrus issued a decree permitting the Jews to return to their homeland and build the second Temple for Yahweh (Ezra 1:1–3). Yet after sixteen years, construction of the Temple had made little headway due to the considerable opposition the Jews faced from local Samaritans.[3] Due to the stagnant progress, God sent His prophet Haggai to provide guidance and strength to the people.

> "Thus says Yahweh of hosts: 'This people says, "*The time has not come to rebuild the temple of Yahweh.*"'" And the word of Yahweh came *through* Haggai the prophet, saying, "*Is it* a time for you yourselves to dwell in your houses that have been paneled *while* this house *is* desolate?" And so then, thus says Yahweh of hosts: '*Consider your ways*! You have sown much but have harvested little. You have eaten without *being* satisfied; *you have drunk without being satiated*; you have worn clothes without *being* warm; the one who earns wages puts it in *a pouch with holes*.' Thus says Yahweh of hosts: '*Consider your ways*! Go up the mountain and bring wood and build the house so that I may be pleased with it and honored,' says Yahweh. 'You have looked for much, and look! *It came* to little; and *when* you brought *it*

---

2 Israel P. Loken, *The Old Testament Prophetic Books: An Introduction* (Maitland, FL: Xulon Press, 2010), 337–338.

3 Randall Price, *Rose Guide to the Temple* (Peabody, MA: Rose Publishing, 2012), 60.

home, I blew it *away.* Why?' *declares* Yahweh of hosts. 'Because my house *is* desolate and you *are* running each to your own house! Therefore, because of you *the* heavens have withheld *the* dew and the earth has withheld its produce. I have called for a drought on the land and the hills, on the grain, the new wine, the olive oil, on what the soil produces, on human beings and wild animals, and on *all their labor.*'" (Hag. 1:2–11)

> But my righteous one will live by faith,
>   and if he shrinks back, my soul is not
>   well pleased with him.
> (Heb. 10:38)

The returned remnants faced strong and relentless opposition from the Samaritans in their pursuit to construct the second Temple. They suffered numerous defeats, which left them in great despair and devastation. In this state of crushing disappointment, the remnants redirected their efforts from Temple construction to tending to their own homes and livelihoods, such as farming. While His people temporarily ceased working on the Temple, God's plan remained. He raised King Darius to assist the remnants in the Temple's construction and ward off the Samaritan opposition.

However, during the cessation, their priorities gradually shifted from the divine tasks which united them as one to individualistic tasks seeking after personal gain. Their hope was now anchored in their own labor rather than in the reconstruction of the second Temple. Just as Deuteronomy 11:16–17 had warned, relentless cycles of droughts, pestilence, and failed harvests plagued them as they turned away from serving God to pursue their own interests. Despite their persistent labor, they lived in dire famine and poverty. Instead of repenting, these struggles in their daily lives further compelled them to prioritize earthly concerns.

God implored the remnants to reflect on their ways as they were once more caught in the cycle of backsliding into sin and endured the torment resulting from those sins. He pleaded with them to seek repentance and ultimately to seek deliverance. God's call, "Consider your ways," was His exhortation for His people to return to and stay on the path of their faith and divine calling. God urged them to live by faith, charging forward without shrinking back.

> Zerubbabel son of Shealtiel, Joshua son of Jehozadak, the high priest, and all the remnant of the people gave heed to the voice of Yahweh their God and to the words of Haggai the prophet, as Yahweh their God had sent him, *and the people feared Yahweh*. And Haggai the messenger of Yahweh spoke to the people with the message of Yahweh, saying, "'I *am* with you' *declares* Yahweh." And Yahweh stirred up the spirit of Zerubbabel son of Shealtiel, governor of Judah, and the spirit of Joshua son of Jehozadak, the high priest, and the spirit of all the remnant of the people. And they came and did *the* work on the house of Yahweh of hosts, their God, on the twenty-fourth day of the sixth month in the second year of King Darius. (Hag. 1:12–15)

Despite a temporary detour, their profound reverence for God drove them to obey His word. God was among them, igniting the spirit of all the people of Judah, boosting and fortifying them. The twenty-three-day gap between the prophecy and the start of work was for planning and preparation. This quick response illustrates their eagerness to resume the Temple's reconstruction. Their fear of God prompted obedience, starting with leaders like Zerubbabel and Joshua and extending to all the remaining people. Their repentance wasn't just a fleeting spiritual experience; it translated into a meaningful change in the direction of their lives.

> In the seventh *month* on the twenty-first day, the word of Yahweh *came through* Haggai the prophet, saying, "Speak now to Zerubbabel son of Shealtiel, governor of Judah, and to Joshua son of Jehozadak, the high priest, and to the remnant of the people, saying . . ." (Hag. 2:1–2)

Speak to the *Israelites*, saying, 'On the fifteenth day of the seventh month, this *shall be* the Feast of Booths for seven days for Yahweh. On the first day there shall be a holy assembly; you must not do any *regular work. For* seven days you must present an offering made by fire to Yahweh. On the eighth day it shall be a holy assembly for you, and you shall present an offering made by fire to Yahweh; it *is* a celebration; you must not do *any regular work.*' (Lev. 23:34–36)

The second prophecy of Haggai, occurring on the seventh day of the Tabernacle Feast, was directed to all the people of Judah who had returned to Jerusalem. This prophesy was about two months after he had spoken to them the first time.

'Who among you *is* left that saw this house in its former glory? How do you see it now? Does it seem like nothing *to you*? 'But now take courage, Zerubbabel,' *declares* Yahweh. 'Take courage, Joshua son of Jehozadak, the high priest, and take courage, all the people of the land,' *declares* Yahweh. 'Do the work, because I *am* with you,' *declares* Yahweh of hosts, 'according to *the promise* that *I covenanted* with you when you came out of Egypt. My spirit *is with you*; do not be afraid.' (Hag. 2:3–5)

The first Temple for Yahweh, built by King Solomon, radiated opulence and grandeur. It was a true masterpiece crafted by the world's finest artisans, adorned with rare materials, including marble, gold, and precious gemstones. The task of rebuilding the Temple couldn't compare to the magnificence of the original. This humbling comparison was disheartening to the remnants building the second Temple. However, in their despair, God came and encouraged them with His faithfulness and kindness, reminding them that His presence would still grace this second Temple, and that its significance went beyond mere physical grandeur.

For thus says Yahweh of hosts: 'Once again, in a little while, I will shake the heavens and the earth and the sea and dry land. I will shake all the nations so that the treasure of all the nations will come, and I will fill this house *with* glory,' says Yahweh of hosts. 'The silver *is* mine and the gold *is* mine,' *declares* Yahweh of hosts. 'The latter glory of this house will be greater than the former,' says Yahweh of hosts, 'and in this place I will give peace' *declares* Yahweh of hosts. (Hag. 2:6–9)

God unveiled His plan to bring about a tumultuous period with empires violently rising and falling amid chaotic clashes and relentless internal wars. He made this revelation to guide His people to understand what was about to happen around them in preparation for the coming of the Messiah, the treasure of all nations. God called the Messiah the treasure of all nations, conveying that His plan for redemption through the Messiah encompassed not just the remnants but also the Gentiles.

This prophecy found its fulfillment in the conquest of the Persian Empire by Alexander the Great, whose sudden death led to his four successors engaging in battles with each other. Two of his successors prevailed but were ultimately subdued by the Roman Empire. During the era of Great Wars, a political unity was achieved through the widespread use of the Greek language and the Roman road system, connecting the capital to its provinces. Many acknowledge that if Christ had been born fifty years earlier, His ministry and the wide spread of His teaching would have been unimaginable.[4]

> On *the* twenty-fourth *day* of the ninth *month*, in the second year of Darius, the word of Yahweh came to the prophet Haggai, saying, "Thus says Yahweh of hosts: 'Ask now the priests *for* a ruling.'" (2:10–11)

Approximately fourteen months after the second prophecy, God once again spoke through His prophet Haggai, addressing the priests first and then Zerubbabel, the governor of Judah. As

---

4 F.F. Bruce, *The Spreading Flame* (Grand Rapids: Eerdmans, 1995), 24–25.

indicated in 2:18, this was yet another feast day on which the Jews laid the foundation of the second Temple.

> If a man carries consecrated meat in the hem of his garment, and his hem touches bread, or stew, or wine, or olive oil, or any kind of food, will it become holy?'" The priests answered, "No." Then Haggai said, "If one who is unclean from contact with a corpse touches any of these, will it become unclean?" The priests answered, "Yes, it will become unclean." Haggai answered and said, "'So *it is with* this people, and *with* this nation before me,' *declares* Yahweh, 'and so *it is with* every kind of work of their hands; and what they offer there *is* unclean. But now, please *consider* from this day forward, before one stone was placed on another in the temple of Yahweh, *from that time when* one came to a heap of twenty *measures*, there were *only* ten, and *when* one came to the wine vat to draw out fifty measures, there were *only* twenty. I struck you with blight, and with plant mildew, and hail, all the work of your hands. But *you did not come back to me*,' *declares* Yahweh. '*Please consider* from this day forward, from the twenty-fourth day of the ninth *month*, from the day that the foundation of Yahweh's temple was laid, *consider*: *Is there* still seed in the store chamber? Do the vine, the fig tree, the pomegranate, and the olive tree still produce nothing? From this day *forward* I will bless *you*.'" (Hag. 2:12–19)

Yahweh taught the priests that holiness cannot be transferred, but impurity can. He highlighted the point that falling into sin is easier than attaining righteousness. God implored His priests to safeguard the purity of their hearts, as this preceded any change in their actions, which could then spread like wildfire in a forest. He recalled the days of sorrow and fruitless labor in their previous sinful state, for God had opposed the people. During these incredibly challenging times, their crop yield fell short of their expectations by half each year. Starting from this moment, He promised to abundantly bless them, ensuring that their labor would no longer be in vain.

The word of Yahweh came to Haggai a second time on the twenty-fourth *day* of the month saying, "Say to Zerubbabel, governor of Judah: I *am* going to shake the heavens and the earth, and I will overthrow the thrones of kingdoms and destroy the military strength of the kingdoms of the nations. I will overthrow chariots and their drivers; horses and their riders will fall, every one by the sword of another! 'On that day,' *declares* Yahweh of hosts, 'I will take you, Zerubbabel son of Shealtiel, my servant,' *declares* Yahweh, 'and I will make you a signet ring, for I have chosen you,' *declares* Yahweh of hosts." (Hag. 2:20–23)

On the same day, Haggai delivered another prophecy. This time, the recipient was Zerubbabel, a descendant of the Davidic line through Solomon, Josiah, and Jehoiachin (1 Chron. 3:15–19). Haggai vividly described to him the shaking of all nations, which would be followed by the arrival of the Messiah "on that day." He assured Zerubbabel that the Messiah would still come through the Davidic lineage. From that point forward, this prophecy was linked to the Messiah, to whom Yahweh refers as His signet ring. In ancient Israel, a signet ring wasn't merely a transmitter of power; it symbolized the very embodiment of the individual wearing it.[5] Christ truly embodied the authority, power, and permanence of Yahweh and came through the Davidic line, as promised to Zerubbabel.

The ABC (Abstract to Brick Concrete)

Feast—General Definition:[6]

- An elaborate and usually abundant meal often accompanied by a ceremony or entertainment; a periodic religious

---

5 Laura Quick, *Dress, Adornment, and the Body in the Hebrew Bible* (Oxford, UK: Oxford University Press, 2021), 43–46.

6 "Feast," Merriam-Webster.com, accessed October 23, 2023, https://www.merriam-webster.com.

observance commemorating an event or honoring a deity, person, or thing.

Feast—Biblical Definition:

- A moment of celebration where His people connect with God, unite as a community, and realign their lives and actions with His will.

The FAST (Focused, Actionable Steps to Take)

During holiday celebrations, strengthen your relationship with God and fellow Christians by nurturing spiritual communion and fostering unity. Consider organizing gatherings with fellow believers to mark the occasion with expressions of joy, love, and kindness rooted in your shared faith in Christ. These heartfelt get-togethers can serve as opportunities for fellowship, prayer, and sharing your spiritual journeys, deepening your sense of community and strengthening the bonds that tie you to both God and your fellow believers.

Example 1: Pamela took the initiative to organize a foot-washing ceremony on Easter for her church community, where they collectively learned about humility and servanthood, drawing inspiration from Christ's example. During this ceremony, all the community members participated and humbly washed one another's feet, symbolizing these virtues and deepening their spiritual bonds.

Example 2: George arranged a Gratitude Circle for Thanksgiving, where the community had the opportunity to practice gratitude and reflect on God's help in their lives. Each person shared what they were thankful for, creating an atmosphere of appreciation, unity, and spiritual growth within the group.

32

Christ Quest, Part 1

Spreading the Gospel Against All Odds—Paul

> *Now* after they *traveled through Amphipolis and Apollonia, they came to Thessalonica, where there was a synagogue of the Jews.* As was his custom, *Paul went in to them and on three Sabbath* days *he discussed with them from the scriptures, explaining and demonstrating that it was necessary* for *the Christ to suffer and to rise from the dead, and* saying, *"This Jesus whom I am proclaiming to you is the Christ." Some of them were persuaded and joined Paul and Silas, and* also *a large number of God-fearing Greeks and not a few of the prominent women.*
>
> Acts 17:1–4

THE APOSTLE PAUL and his companions boldly proclaimed the gospel to the people of Thessalonica. While this was well-received by the Greeks, it sparked jealousy among the Jews. Since his ministry team operated within the synagogue, the Gentile converts were situated within the context and jurisdiction of the Jewish community. As the body of Gentile converts grew within the community, the Jews became increasingly aware of Paul's ministry. Most of the Gentile converts in Thessalonica were "God-fearing Greeks." This term encompasses a wide spectrum of Gentile adherents, from full conversion to showing amicable support for the Jewish community.[1]

> But the Jews were filled with jealousy and, taking along some worthless men from the rabble in the marketplace and forming a mob, threw the city into an uproar. And attacking Jason's house, they were looking for *them* to bring them out to the popular assembly. And *when they* did not find them, they dragged Jason and some brothers before the city officials, shouting, "These *people* who have stirred up trouble *throughout* the world have come here also, whom Jason has entertained as guests! These *people are* all acting contrary to the decrees of Caesar, saying there is another king, Jesus!" And they threw the crowd into confusion, and the city officials who heard these *things*. And *after* taking money as security from Jason and the rest, they released them. (Acts 17:5–9)

Paul, a Jewish man, faced not just opposition but also intense jealousy and hostility from many unconverted Jews. While they openly cited their disagreement with Jesus being the Christ as the cause of their hostility, the intensity of their animosity went beyond what could be explained by a mere disagreement with his teachings. The underlying tension stemmed from their understandable sense of unease and jealousy about the changes his ministry introduced. Subconsciously, they recognized that Paul was fulfilling a role they believed should be theirs—leading Gentiles in worshipping God. The Jews felt that their own mission was unfolding before their eyes without their active participation, and this complexity of emotions likely contributed to the misdirected hostility.

---

1 James P. Ware, *The Mission of the Church in Paul's Letter to the Philippians in the Context of Ancient Judaism* (Leiden, The Netherlands: Brill, 2005), 32–43.

A group of unbelieving Jews rounded up a band of notorious ruffians, known for their disorderly conduct, to stand with them in their opposition to Paul and his company. They staged a protest against the missionaries in the city, culminating in a daring attack on the house of Paul's generous host, Jason. Unable to locate Paul, they seized Jason and several other Christians, forcibly bringing them before the city officials.

The Jews accused the Christians of rebelling against the Roman Empire by alleging their allegiance to another king, Jesus. The individuals involved with Paul's ministry were held legally responsible by the city officials and had to pay a "security." The word "security" in Acts 17:9 originates from the Greek term *hikanos*, often used in legal contexts for bail.[2] This peace bond was intended to ensure they would not repeat the same offense. Thus, they avoided being sent to the Roman provincial magistrates on charges of treason. City officials took this security measure in response to the serious allegation of treason to demonstrate their loyalty to Rome. To maintain public order, they prioritized crowd appeasement over the pursuit of justice.

> Now the brothers sent away both Paul and Silas at once, during the night, to Berea. *They* went into the synagogue of the Jews *when they* arrived. Now these were more open-minded than those in Thessalonica. *They* accepted the message with all eagerness, examining the scriptures every day *to see* if these *things* were so. Therefore many of them believed, and not a few of the prominent Greek women and men. (17:10–12)

The newly converted believers in Thessalonica grew worried about the increasing hostility from the local Jewish community toward Paul and his missionary team. Under the cover of night, they aided them in leaving the city to avoid any potential harm

---

2   Matthew D. Aernie, *Forensic Language and the Day of the Lord Motif in Second Thessalonians 1 and the Effects on the Meaning of the Text* (Eugene, OR: Wipf & Stock, 2011), 63–65.

from the Jews. These believers guided them to a nearby satellite village called Berea, offering protection and keeping them out of the reach of the local Jewish community.

Berea was a small farming town nestled in the foothills of Mount Bermium in Southern Macedonia. In contrast to the Thessalonians, the people of Berea were open-minded in their acceptance of the gospel. Berea was close to Pella, the hometown of Alexander the Great and a center of Hellenism.[3] As a result, Bereans were familiar with Hellenic philosophy, which played a significant role in shaping their perspective. Hellenism, known for its tolerance toward new religious and philosophical ideas, prepared them to receive the gospel readily.[4] This receptive attitude of the Bereans was advantageous for Paul's missionary work, as it facilitated a more fruitful and welcoming environment for his teachings.

> But when the Jews from Thessalonica found out that the message of God had been proclaimed by Paul in Berea also, they came there too, inciting and stirring up the crowds. So then the brothers sent Paul away at once to go to the sea, and both Silas and Timothy remained there. Those who conducted Paul brought *him* as far as Athens, and *after* receiving an order for Silas and Timothy that they should come to him as soon as possible, they went away. (Acts 17:13–15)

Berea, also known as Veria, was located approximately fifty miles southwest of Thessalonica.[5] A group of Jews from Thessalonica embarked on a two-day journey to Berea with the intent to capture and harm Paul for spreading the gospel. Neither the

---

3 John R. Miles, *A Dictionary of Scripture Geography* (Manchester, England: Thomas Johnson, 1852), 66.

4 Jacob Neusner and Bruce Chilton, *Religious Tolerance in World Religions* (West Conshohocken, PA: Templeton Foundation Press, 2008), 47–49.

5 James S. Jeffers, *The Greco-Roman World of the New Testament Era* (Downers Grove, IL: InterVarsity Press, 1999), 281–282.

harsh terrain nor the scorching heat deterred them from their relentless pursuit. The entire expedition likely spanned about a week or two, with four grueling days spent walking to and from Berea. Their sinister determination became apparent even to the people in Berea, who promptly sent Paul far away to Athens, a three-day voyage by sea, to ensure his safety, preventing him from falling into their hands.[6]

> For *you* yourselves know, brothers, our reception with you, that it was not in vain, but *after we* had already suffered and been mistreated in Philippi, just as you know, we had the courage in our God to speak to you the gospel of God amid much opposition. For our exhortation *is* not from error or from impurity or with deceit, but just as we have been approved by God to be entrusted with the gospel, thus we speak, not as pleasing people but God, who examines our hearts. *For never* did we come with a word of flattery, just as you know, nor with a pretext of greediness (God *is* witness), nor seeking glory from people, neither from you nor from others. *Although we could have insisted on our own importance* as apostles of Christ, yet we became infants in your midst, like a nursing mother cherishes her own children. Longing for you in this way, we determined to share with you not only the gospel of God but also our own souls, because you had become dear to us. (1 Thess. 2:1–8)

After his missionary work in Thessalonica, Paul faced a situation that required him to write letters to the Thessalonians. In these letters, he sought to address misunderstandings and unfounded allegations that had arisen against him. These issues were not only affecting his ministry but also undermining the gospel and the early Christian community. First, he needed to clarify that his imprisonment in Philippi resulted from spreading the gospel. He emphasized that their ministry aimed to please God,

---

6 Paton J. Gloag, *A Critical and Exegetical Commentary on the Acts of the Apostles* (Edinburgh, Scotland: T & T Clark, 1870), 142.

not people, with a pure desire to serve Him, devoid of hidden motives. He also stressed that their ministry had God's approval, and the gospel they preached was directly from Him, ensuring the accuracy of their teaching.

> For you remember, brothers, our labor and hardship: working by night and day in order not to be a burden to any of you, we proclaimed to you the gospel of God. You *are* witnesses, and *so is* God, how devoutly and righteously and blamelessly we became to you who believe, just as you know how *we treated* each one of you, like a father his own children, exhorting and consoling you and insisting that you live in a manner worthy of God, who calls you to his own kingdom and glory. (1 Thess. 2:9–12)

In the first century, philosophers known as sophists traveled from city to city, charging fees for teaching on a range of topics, including philosophy, religion, and politics. This practice established a marketplace for the exchange of philosophical ideas and knowledge during that period.[7] In that cultural context, it would have been customary for the apostle Paul to be paid for teaching the gospel. Nonetheless, he gave up the right to avoid burdening the converts. Instead, he worked tirelessly as a tentmaker, using his own hands to support both himself and his ministry (Acts 18:3). His reference to "night and day" (1 Thess. 2:9) indicates that he began his work before the break of dawn and continued laboring late into the night each day. This rigorous schedule encompassed his dual role as a tentmaker and preacher of the gospel.

> Because of this we also give thanks to God constantly, that *when you* received God's word *that you heard* from us, you accepted *it* not *as the* word of men, but as *it* truly is, *the* word of God, which also is at work in you who believe. For you became imitators, brothers, of the churches of God *which* are in Judea in Christ Jesus, because you also suffered the same *things* at the hands of

---

7 Bill Cooke, *Dictionary of Atheism, Skepticism, & Humanism* (Amherst, NY: Prometheus, 2009), 495–497.

your own people, just as *they* themselves *did* also at the hands of the Jews, who killed both the Lord Jesus and the prophets, and who persecuted us, and *who are* not pleasing to God and *are* opposed to all people, hindering us from speaking to the Gentiles in order that they may be saved, so that *they* always fill up their sins. But wrath has come upon them to the end. (1 Thess. 2:13–16)

Shortly after embracing the gospel, the Thessalonians began to experience persecution. Despite these trials, their unwavering faith remained steadfast. Paul astutely praised them by drawing a parallel between their resilience and that of the Judean Christians, who endured prolonged persecution. In 2:15–16, Paul pronounced divine judgment upon the Jewish oppressors of the gospel. This specific group, often hailing from privileged social backgrounds, strongly opposed the gospel and subjected the followers of Christ, whether Jews or Gentiles, to severe persecution.[8]

But *when* we were made orphans by separation from you, brothers, for *a short time* (in face, not in heart), *we were* even more eager with great desire to see your face, because we wanted to come to you—I, Paul, *on more than one occasion*—and Satan hindered us. For who *is* our hope or joy or crown of boasting? *Is it* not even you, in the presence of our Lord Jesus at his coming? For you are our glory and joy. (2:17–20)

Paul held the Thessalonians close to his heart, considering them his hope, joy, and a source of pride. In his role as the spiritual shepherd of this Christian community, he bore the weighty responsibility for their well-being and spiritual growth. Even amid the trials, they continued to flourish, standing as a testament to his missionary excellence. He depicted Christ's return as a reason for celebration for them rather than a day of fearful judgment, as they now belong to Christ and not to this world.

---

8 Thomas R. Schreiner, *Paul, Apostle of God's Glory in Christ: A Pauline Theology* (Downers Grove, IL: InterVarsity Press, 2001), 474–475.

This message, filled with hope for His return, was intended to praise their faith and commitment.

> Therefore *when we* could bear *it* no longer, we determined to be left behind in Athens alone, and we sent Timothy, our brother and fellow worker for God in the gospel of Christ, in order to strengthen and to encourage you about your faith, *so that* no one would be shaken by these afflictions. For *you* yourselves know that we are appointed for this, for indeed when we were with you we told you beforehand that we were about to be afflicted, just as indeed it happened, and you know. Because of this, I also, *when I* could endure *it* no longer, sent in order to know your faith, lest somehow the tempter tempted you and our labor should be in vain. (1 Thess. 3:1–5)

> Indeed, all those who want to live in a godly manner in Christ Jesus will be persecuted. (2 Tim. 3:12)

When Paul noted the steadfast devotion of the Thessalonians to Christ, he was certain that persecution was on the horizon. Referring to 3:12, he conveyed to them that all followers of Christ would endure persecution. He prepared them to take persecution as a confirmation of their genuine faith rather than a reason to lose it. When this forewarned persecution began, it led to his departure, leaving the new converts to grapple with adversity.

Even after his expulsion from Thessalonica, Paul continued his dedicated ministry to the new Christian community. As the persecution intensified, he grew concerned about whether the new believers might choose to renounce their faith in Christ. On this account, Paul dispatched Timothy, his right-hand support, to revisit them, demonstrating the extent of his care for the survival of their faith.

> But now, *because* Timothy has come to us from you and has brought good news to us of your faith and love, and that *you always think kindly of us*, desiring to see us just as also we *desire to see* you, because of this, brothers, we have been comforted because of you in all our distress and affliction

through your faith, because now we live, if you stand firm in the Lord. (1 Thess. 3:6–8)

Paul endured agonizing months of uncertainty, not knowing whether the Thessalonian believers had lost their faith. When Timothy finally returned, he brought overwhelmingly positive news: the Thessalonian believers stood strong in their faith and love despite the escalating persecution. Amid his ministry trials and afflictions in Corinth, Paul found profound solace in this news. The sight of the Thessalonian believers, unwavering in the face of relentless adversity, served as a testament to the success of his ministry. It reassured him that his tireless efforts and sacrifices were far from in vain.

> For what thanks can we repay to God concerning you, because of all the joy *with* which we rejoice because of you before our God, nights and days praying beyond all measure that *we* may see your face and complete what is lacking in your faith? Now *may* our God and Father himself and our Lord Jesus direct our way to you, and *may* the Lord *cause* you to increase and to abound in love for one another and for all, just as also we *do* for you, so that your hearts may be established blameless in holiness before our God and Father at the coming of our Lord Jesus with all his saints. (3:9–13)

> A new commandment I [Christ] give to you: that you love one another—just as I have loved you, that you also love one another. By this everyone will know that you are my disciples—if you have love for one another. (John 13:34–35)

In First Thessalonians 3:10, the phrase "beyond all measure" translates the Hebrew word *huper*, an exceptionally strong version of "exceedingly." It may be translated as "very, very exceedingly," emphasizing the idea of something being extremely or overwhelmingly beyond normal measures or expectations.[9] Paul engaged in

---

9 Charles C. Ryrie, *First & Second Thessalonians: Everyman's Bible Commentary* (Chicago: Moody Publishers, 2001), 48–50.

this intense level of prayer because he desired to reunite with them so he could guide their spiritual growth. His ministry wasn't only about salvation; it also involved nurturing their faith to keep it strong and complete.

His prayer was also for the Thessalonian believers to continue practicing abounding love for one another and to extend this love to everyone around them, including their persecutors and enemies. This supplication was rooted in his understanding that their love and unity in Christ made them righteous and thus acceptable to God.

Amid persecution, Paul reminded the Thessalonian believers of Christ's return, which served as a source of hope and encouragement. It assured them that their struggles held meaning and that, with it, a time of peace, justice, and the fulfillment of God's promises awaited. This message would have brought them comfort and courage in challenging times.

The ABC (Abstract to Brick Concrete)

Persecution—General Definition:[10]

- Being made to suffer because of belief.

Persecution—Biblical Definition:

- An acknowledgment from the world of an individual's fulfillment of their divine mission.

The FAST (Focused, Actionable Steps to Take)

1. Persecution often seeks to divide and weaken the faith community. By helping each other, Christians demonstrate unity and solidarity, sending a powerful message to those who would seek to persecute them.

---

10 "Persecution," Merriam-Webster.com, accessed October 23, 2023, https://www.merriam-webster.com.

Example: Ben and Rick found themselves in a challenging situation when their non-Christian parents learned about their consistent church attendance. Despite their parents' strong disapproval, they continued to practice their faith. As a result, their parents suddenly cut off their financial support, making it difficult for them to socialize with their church friends as they used to and also hindering their participation in youth group events due to financial constraints. Their friend from church, Ann, called to check on them and learned about their situation. Upon finding out that their parents had cut their financial support, she offered to provide them with rides to church services and youth group events. This assistance allowed them to stay connected with their faith community despite the financial hardships.

2. Support your fellow Christians who are facing persecution by standing with them. Offer them spiritual guidance, practical help, and advocacy in their time of need.

   Example: Lisa's supervisor, Terry, is against the gospel and deliberately assigns her to work on Sundays whenever there's an opportunity. This is because Terry is aware of her strong Christian faith and commitment to attending church services. Yolanda, a fellow Christian who understands her situation, has been incredibly supportive. Every Sunday, she records their church's worship service and sends it to Lisa. This ensures that even when she can't attend in person due to her work schedule, she can still participate in the worship and stay connected with the faith community.

33

Christ Quest, Part 2

Faith, Hope, and the Second Coming—Paul

Finally therefore, brothers, we ask you and appeal to you **in the Lord Jesus** *that, just as you have received from us how it is necessary for you to live and to please God, just as indeed you are living, that you progress even more. For you know what commands we gave to you through the Lord Jesus. For this is the will of God, your sanctification:* **that** *you abstain from sexual immorality;* **that** *each of you know how to possess his own vessel in sanctification and honor, not in lustful passion, just as also the Gentiles who do not know God; not to transgress and to exploit his brother in the matter, because the Lord* **is** *the one who avenges concerning all these* **things***, just as also we told you beforehand and testified solemnly. For God did not call us to impurity, but in holiness. Therefore the one who rejects* **this** *is not rejecting man, but God,* **who** *also gives his Holy Spirit to you.*

First Thessalonians 4:1–8

THE APOSTLE PAUL encouraged the Thessalonians to live according to God's will, explaining that their sanctification involved practical steps, such as abstaining from sexual immorality. The sexual immorality mentioned in First Thessalonians 4:3, derived from the Greek word *porneia*, covers a wide range of lust-driven behaviors, spanning from fornication, prostitution, orgies, carousing, and extending even to bestiality.[1] The Cabeiri served as the fertility gods and patrons of Thessalonica. Their worship involved sexually immoral practices, such as grotesque phallic rituals.[2] Participating in sexually immoral acts was a form of idolatrous worship dedicated to the Cabeiri. In a culture endorsing such practices, particularly the worship of the Cabeiri, Paul urged them to stand apart from the sin and actively pursue Christ's standards.[3]

> But concerning brotherly love, I do not need to write to you, for you yourselves are taught by God to love one another, for indeed you are practicing it toward all the brothers in all of Macedonia. But we urge you, brothers, to progress even more, and to aspire to live a quiet life, and to attend to *your own business*, and to work with your hands, just as we commanded you, so that you may live decently toward those outside, and may have need of nothing. (4:9–12)

The phrase "taught by God" in 4:9 is rooted in the Greek word *theodidaktos* and signifies divine interpersonal wisdom for unity among fellow believers in Christ.[4] It extends to encouraging

---

1 Charles A. Wanamaker, *The Epistles to the Thessalonians: A Commentary on the Greek Text* (Grand Rapids: Eerdmans, 1990), 151–152.

2 Andy Johnson, *1 and 2 Thessalonians* (Grand Rapids: Eerdmans, 2016), 107–108; Richard N. Longenecker, *Patterns of Discipleship in the New Testament* (Grand Rapids: Eerdmans, 1996), 103–107.

3 Dennis L. Merritt, *The Cry of Merlin: Jung, the Prototypical Ecopsychologist* (Carmel, CA: Fisher King Press, 2012), 167.

4 Stuart C. Devenish, *Seeing and Believing: The Eye of Faith in a Visual Culture* (Eugene, OR: Wipf & Stock, 2012), 68.

kindness and compassion, even toward unbelievers within their community. This principle mirrors Christ's teaching that His disciples would be set apart from the world by their unconditional love and servitude toward one another (John 13:34–35).

In first-century Greco-Roman society, manual labor was deemed lowly. Thessalonian converts, mainly from the working class and slaves, misunderstood their freedom in Christ as releasing them from work obligations. This misconception led them to forsake labor and depend on others for their needs. Paul encouraged them to return to work, reintegrate into society, and manifest Christian virtues such as integrity, kindness, and compassion in their societal roles. He aimed to reframe labor from being a degrading obligation to an opportunity to serve as the light of the world, manifesting the glory of God.

> Now we do not want you to be ignorant, brothers, concerning those who have fallen asleep, so that you will not grieve as also the rest, who have no hope. For if we believe that Jesus died and rose *again*, thus also God will bring those who have fallen asleep through Jesus together with him. For this we say to you by the word of the Lord, that we who are alive, who remain until the Lord's coming, will not possibly precede those who have fallen asleep. (1 Thess. 4:13–15)

The new believers in Thessalonica eagerly awaited the return of Christ, grappling with the concern that they might pass away beforehand. Their concern also revolved around their loved ones who had died before the second coming of Christ, fearing that these dear ones might not enter the kingdom with them. Paul reassured them that those who passed away before His return, would be brought back to life through Christ. They would all share in the Great Feast, entering the kingdom of heaven, just as Christ had promised.

> For the Lord himself will descend from heaven with a shout of command, with the voice of the archangel and with the trumpet of God, and the dead in Christ will rise first. Then we who are

alive, who remain, will be snatched away at the same time together with them in the clouds for a meeting with the Lord in the air, and thus we will be together with the Lord always. Therefore comfort one another with these words. (1 Thess. 4:16–18)

Paul painted a vivid image of the glorious return of Christ. He described how Christ would descend from the heavens amid a commanding shout, the resounding voice of the archangel, and the powerful blast of God's trumpet. Whether his beloved followers were already deceased or still alive, all would be gathered into the arms of Christ. From that moment on, they would be in the timeless communion with Christ. Paul instructed them to find comfort in these words, encouraging each other with the hope of this eternal life with Christ.

> Now concerning the times and the seasons, brothers, you have no need *of anything* to be written to you for *you* yourselves well know that the day of the Lord is coming in the *same* way as a thief in the night. Whenever they say "Peace and security," then sudden destruction will overtake them like the birth pains of *a pregnant woman*, and they will not possibly escape. But you, brothers, are not in the darkness, so that the day should catch you like a thief, for you are all sons of light and sons of day. We are not of the night nor of darkness. (1 Thess. 5:1–5)

During the 200-year Pax Romana, characterized by unprecedented peace and prosperity, the government promoted the propaganda "peace and security" on various platforms, including political speeches, coins, and monuments. People of that era, including the Thessalonians, attributed their prosperity and security directly to the Pax Romana.[5] Paul noted the deceptive nature of the propaganda, emphasizing that the return of Christ will shatter this false illusion. He warned nonbelievers that the day of

---

5 Jeffrey A.D. Weima, "'Peace and Security' (1 Thess 5:3): Prophetic Warning or Political Propaganda?" *New Testament Studies*, Vol. 58.3 (2012), 331–359.

judgment will be upon them like a thief in the night. However, those who follow Christ will be spared from God's wrath, as He has set them apart to belong to Him, distinct from those affiliated with the world.

> So then, we must not sleep like the rest, but must be on the alert and be self-controlled. For those who sleep, sleep at night, and those who get drunk, are drunk at night. But *because* we are of the day, we must be sober, *by* putting on the breastplate of faith and love and *as* a helmet the hope of salvation, because God did not appoint us for wrath, but for the obtaining of salvation through our Lord Jesus Christ, who died for us, so that whether we are awake or asleep, we will live at the same time with him. Therefore encourage one another and build up *each other*, just as indeed you are doing. (1 Thess. 5:6–11)

Paul used military language to prompt Christians to equip themselves for the ongoing spiritual warfare, which will only intensify until the return of Christ. To gear up for the battle, he instructed them to don a helmet of hope for salvation and a breastplate for faith and love. Hope is a robust, future-oriented confidence driving one towards desired goals. Keeping hope in Christ means aligning one's goals, motivations, and affections with His standards. Faith is an unwavering trust and belief in God's covenants and divine characteristics. Love is a unifying force bringing believers together to achieve common goals of glorifying God. Paul again encouraged them to continue building each other up, fostering a community of genuine care and love.

> Now we ask you, brothers, to respect those who labor among you and rule over you in the Lord and admonish you, and to esteem them beyond all measure in love, because of their work. Be at peace among yourselves. (1 Thess. 5:12–13)

In the face of the Pharisees and Sadducees' derision, regarding the early church leaders as "uneducated and untrained" (Acts

4:13), Paul urges the church members to respect those who tirelessly minister to them day and night.[6] Paul emphasizes an extraordinary level of respect using the phrase "beyond all measure," translating the Hebrew expression *huper*. This prescribed level of respect is exceptionally strong, akin to "very, very exceedingly."[7]

> We urge you, brothers, admonish the disorderly, console the discouraged, help the sick, and be patient toward all *people*. See to it that no one pays back evil for evil to anyone, but always pursue good toward one another and toward all *people*. (1 Thess. 5:14–15)

Paul urged the Thessalonians to support one another by instructing those who deviated from God's ways, comforting the disheartened, and aiding those facing challenging circumstances. He also guided them not to retaliate when faced with wrongdoing. Instead, they were to choose the path of goodness toward one another and everyone else. He strived to foster a strong, harmonious community among the Thessalonians.

> Rejoice always, pray constantly, give thanks in everything; for this *is* the will of God for you in Christ Jesus. Do not quench the Spirit. Do not despise prophecies, but examine all *things*; hold fast to *what is* good. Abstain from every form of evil. (5:16–22)

Paul composed a series of staccato bursts to emphasize his teaching on individual spiritual development.

The teachings included the importance of rejoicing, praying, and giving thanks in all circumstances, avoiding the discouragement of fellow believers, and carefully examining prophecies before dismissing them. He also taught them to

---

6 John Phillips, *Exploring 1 & 2 Thessalonians: An Expository Commentary* (Grand Rapids: Kregel, 2005), 139.

7 Charles C. Ryrie, *First & Second Thessalonians: Everyman's Bible Commentary* (Chicago: Moody Publishers, 2001), 48–50.

follow teachings aligned with the Scriptures and reject those that deviate from them.

> Now may the God of peace himself sanctify you completely, and may your spirit and soul and body be kept complete, blameless at the coming of our Lord Jesus Christ. The one who calls you *is* faithful, who also will do *this*.
>
> Brothers, pray for us. Greet all the brothers with a holy kiss. I adjure you by the Lord, have this letter read aloud to all the brothers. The grace of our Lord Jesus Christ *be* with you. (1 Thess. 5:23–28)

Paul wrapped up his letter by praying for the Thessalonians' complete sanctification—asking that they be set apart from worldly influences and consecrated entirely to God's service. In 5:23 Paul discloses is view on the fundamental composition of humanity—a trichotomous constitution encompassing spirit, soul, and body. He underscored that God's sanctifying work pertains to the entire person, not merely the spirit.

He also encouraged the Thessalonian believers to treat each other like family, exchanging warm greetings with holy kisses. His instruction to read the letter aloud demonstrates the value he placed on communal learning. Paul concluded with a blessing, wishing them the grace of Christ.

The ABC (Abstract to Brick Concrete)

Hope—General Definition:[8]

- A desire accompanied by expectation of or belief in fulfillment.

Hope—Biblical Definition:

- A robust, future-oriented confidence in Christ driving one toward their desired goals.

---

[8] "Hope," Merriam-Webster.com, accessed October 23, 2023, https://www.merriam-webster.com.

The FAST (Focused, Actionable Steps to Take)

Align your aspirations with Christ's teachings for a purposeful life. Regularly reflect on your goals, assess progress in line with Scripture, and make adjustments. Dedicate time to read and contemplate the teachings of the Bible. Set aside moments for prayer and meditation, seeking guidance and aligning aspirations with God's will.

Example 1: Every Friday, Stephanie reflects on her goals in her journal, intertwining her thoughts with prayers for divine guidance. She ensures her aspirations align with God's will by reading the Scriptures daily and adjusting her goals based on the teachings of the Scriptures.

Example 2: Max ensures that the media he consumes aligns with Christ's teachings and values. This intentional evaluation helps him consistently align his life goals with these principles.

34

The First Gospel Messenger—Anna

When the days of their purification were completed according to the law of Moses, they brought him up to Jerusalem to present him *to the Lord (just as it is written in the law of the Lord, "Every male that opens the womb will be called holy to the Lord") and to offer a sacrifice according to what was stated in the law of the Lord, "a pair of turtledoves or two young pigeons."*

Luke 2:22–24

But when the fullness of time came, God sent out his Son, born of a woman, born under the law, in order that he might redeem those under the law, in order that we might receive the adoption.

Galatians 4:4–5

THE PURIFICATION ritual Jesus underwent demonstrates His solidarity with His people, as highlighted in 4:4–5. He was born under the law to redeem those bound by it. As the law of Moses states, following the birth of a son, a purification and dedication ceremony must take place, requiring the offering of a male lamb and a dove (Lev. 12:6–7). The law permitted those unable to afford a lamb to offer a pair of doves (12:8), earning it the name "the offering of the poor."[1] Due to their humble financial state, Joseph and Mary presented the offering of the poor for the purification ritual.

> Behold, there was a man in Jerusalem *whose name was* Simeon, and this man *was* righteous and devout, looking forward to the consolation of Israel, and the Holy Spirit was upon him. It had been revealed to him by the Holy Spirit *that he would* not see death before he would see the Lord's Christ. And he came in the Spirit into the temple, and when the parents brought in the child Jesus so that they could do for him according to what was customary under the law, he took him in *his* arms and praised God and said . . . (Luke 2:25–28)

Simeon was a pious man promised by the Holy Spirit that he would see Christ before his death. He was prompted by the Spirit to visit the Temple when Jesus' parents brought Him for the purification ritual. It was there that Simeon encountered the long-awaited Messiah in Mary's arms. He felt a sense of peace, expressing his readiness to depart now that he had finally met the Messiah he had eagerly awaited his entire life.

> "Now dismiss your slave in peace, Lord,
>   according to your word.
> For my eyes have seen your salvation
>   that you have prepared in the presence of all the peoples,
> a light for revelation to the Gentiles,
>   and glory to your people Israel."

> And his father and mother were astonished at what was said about him. Simeon blessed them and said to his mother Mary,

---

[1] William Barclay, *The Gospel of Luke* (Louisville: Westminster John Knox Press, 2001), 30.

"Behold, this child is appointed for the fall and rise of many in Israel, and for a sign that is opposed—and a sword will pierce your own soul also, so that the thoughts of many hearts will be revealed!" (Luke 2:29–35)

> Arise, shine! For your light has come,
> and the glory of Yahweh has risen on you.
> (Isa. 60:1)

Simeon held Christ gently in his arms, speaking with wisdom and knowledge inspired by the Holy Spirit. His prophecy described Christ's mission: saving the Gentiles through the Israelites, thereby honoring them with God's glory. He also prophesied that His ministry would polarize the nation of Israel. This division would expose the true intentions of religious leaders, such as the Pharisees, Sadducees, and Herodians. Despite their outward righteousness, their hearts would betray a deeper presence of transgression as some opposed Christ, leading to their downfall, while others who embraced His message found salvation. Simeon also painted a vivid picture of the soul-piercing anguish Mary would endure, bearing the heart-wrenching sorrow of witnessing her beloved son's rejection and affliction.

> There was a prophetess, Anna the daughter of Phanuel of the tribe of Asher (she was advanced *in years*, having lived with *her* husband seven years *after her marriage*, and herself *as* a widow up to eighty-four years) who did not depart from the temple with fastings and prayers, serving night and day. At *that* same hour she approached *and* began to give thanks to God, and to speak about him to all those who were waiting for the redemption of Jerusalem. (Luke 2:36–38)

Anna, known for her devotion as a prophetess, served within the Temple precincts. Following her husband's early passing, she dedicated the rest of her life to serving Yahweh. At 105 years old, she encountered Jesus at the Temple, where God also revealed to her that He was their long-awaited Messiah.[2] Recognizing that God's salvation, in the form of Christ, had come, Anna poured out profound thanks to God. Anna joyfully proclaimed the Messiah's arrival, with those in Jerusalem eagerly awaiting Him. Anna's proclamation bestowed upon her the honorable title of the first gospel evangelist in history, heralding the message of Christ.

> When they had completed everything according to the law of the Lord, they returned to Galilee, to their own town of Nazareth. The child was growing and becoming strong, filled with wisdom, and the favor of God was upon him. (Luke 2:39–40)

Joseph and Mary exemplified piety by faithfully following the Law of Moses. After fulfilling their obligations, the family returned to their rural hometown, Nazareth. It was a hamlet community sustained by family-owned farms and local quarries.[3] Here in the serene countryside, Jesus matured, gaining strength, wisdom, and divine favor. Despite the extraordinary events surrounding the presentation at the Temple, His childhood bore no immediate earth-shattering changes.

> And his parents went every year to Jerusalem for the feast of the Passover. (2:41)

The Holy Temple in Jerusalem was 70 miles south of Nazareth, demanding a challenging walk of four to six days each way.[4] Their annual attendance at the Great Passover feast again demonstrates their steadfast commitment to following the Mosaic Laws.

---

2 Robert H. Stein, *Luke: An Exegetical and Theological Exposition of Holy Scripture* (Nashville: B&H Publishing Group, 1992), 113–119.

3 Ken R. Dark, *Archaeology of Jesus' Nazareth* (Oxford, UK: Oxford University Press, 2023), 140–146.

4 Walter A. Elwell and Philip W. Comfort, eds., *Tyndale Bible Dictionary* (Wheaton, IL: Tyndale House Publishers, 2001. 1272.

The ABC (Abstract to Brick Concrete)

Evangelism—General Definition:[5]

- The winning or revival of personal commitment to Christ.

Evangelism—Biblical Definition:

- A joyful proclamation of the message that salvation has come through Christ.

The FAST (Focused, Actionable Steps to Take)

Evangelism in our daily lives encompasses both our words and actions, demonstrating the transformative power of Christ. Setting specific and practical goals is key to devising effective strategies and executing daily evangelism.

Example 1: Mason commits herself to distributing six gospel pamphlets monthly within her college. Regularly, during breaks or after classes, she engages with fellow students and colleagues, offering them pamphlets containing messages of hope and faith. Her goal is to consistently share the gospel and connect with individuals, aiming to inspire and uplift them through the literature she shares.

Example 2: Tory posts three Christian messages per week on her social media platforms. Every Monday, Wednesday, and Friday, she shares Bible verses, personal reflections on faith, and stories of God's impact in her life.

Example 3: Jordan sets a personal goal to invite a non-Christian friend or acquaintance to his church every three months. He identifies potential individuals within his circle and extends a warm invitation, sharing details about the church's events and welcoming atmosphere.

---

5 "Evangelism," Merriam-Webster.com, accessed October 23, 2023, https://www.merriam-webster.com.

35

Behold!

Unveiling the Son of God —Jesus of Nazareth

When he [Christ] was twelve years old, they went up according to the custom of the feast. And after the days were completed, while they were returning, the boy Jesus stayed behind in Jerusalem. His parents did not know it, but believing him to be in the group of travelers, they went on a day's journey. They began searching for him among their relatives and their acquaintances, and when they did not find him, they returned to Jerusalem to search for him.

Luke 2:42–45

THIS IS THE ONLY biblical story depicting Jesus' childhood, connecting His presentation at the Temple as an infant to His later adult ministry. It portrays a remarkable occurrence that unfolded after their observance of the Passover festival in the Holy Temple.

Following the feast in Jerusalem, Joseph and Mary, along with numerous travelers, were part of a caravan returning to the Galilee area. As the day drew to a close following their long journey on foot, the family noticed that Jesus was missing. In the grip of gut-wrenching terror, they rushed back to Jerusalem to find Him. The fear of failing in their divine mission to care for Jesus, the Messiah entrusted to them by God, and the unbearable dread of losing their beloved child flooded their hearts and minds with anguish. After a frantic search, they found Jesus engaged in conversations among religious leaders in the Temple, sharing profound insights and sagacity. After searching every street and corner in Jerusalem to no avail, they returned to the Temple in their relentless search for young Jesus. There, they found Jesus engaged in discussions with religious leaders, sharing an astonishing level of insight.

> It happened that after three days they found him in the temple *courts*, sitting in the midst of the teachers and listening to them and asking them *questions*. And all who heard him were amazed at his insight and *his* answers. And *when they* saw him, they were astounded and his mother said to him, "Child, why have you done this to us? Look, your father and I have been searching for you anxiously!" And he said to them, "*Why* were you searching for me? Did you not know that it was necessary *for* me to be in the *house* of my Father?" (Luke 2:46–49)

The word "amazed," used in 2:47, comes from the Greek medical term *existemi*. This term stems from *ek*, meaning out, and *histemi*, meaning to stand, which in Greek implies a flight of the soul from the body.[1] This term captures the profound awe that seized the hearts of religious leaders and elders at the Temple upon encountering His divine wisdom—an experience surpassing earthly understanding.[2] This divine ministry of young Jesus

---

1 Verlyn D. Verbrugge, *New International Dictionary of New Testament Theology: Abridged Edition* (Grand Rapids: Zondervan Academic, 2000), 175–176.

2 Michael A. Rinella, *Pharmakon: Plato, Drug Culture, and Identity in Ancient Athens* (Lanham, MD: Lexington Books, 2010), 36–37.

to the Temple authorities and elders surprised His earthly parents. Their reaction indicates that Jesus lived a typical human life in Nazareth, displaying ordinary growth in the physical, mental, social, and spiritual dimensions. Despite His divine nature, He humbly embraced every aspect of human experience, walking the earth among the people He had created.

Upon finding Him, a rush of emotions flooded through Mary—a mix of relief tinged with hints of terror, panic, and frustration. Her maternal instincts and concern for her family's well-being took precedence over His divine ministry. She reproached Him, pointing out the great distress He had brought upon His parents. However, when Mary referred to his earthly father, Jesus promptly identified the Holy One as his true Father, designating the Holy Temple as his home. He reaffirmed to her His divine calling to serve God, stating that His primary responsibility lay with God rather than His earthly family. This passage illustrates the evolving aspect of His identity as He began to assume His role as the Son of God as the time for his ministry approached.

> They did not understand the statement that he spoke to them. And he went down with them and came to Nazareth, and was submitting to them. And his mother treasured all these things in her heart.
>
> And Jesus was advancing in wisdom and stature and in favor with God and *with* people. (Luke 2:50–52)
>
> Do not think that I have come to destroy the law or the prophets. I have not come to destroy *them* but to fulfill *them*. (Matt. 5:17)

Jesus plainly declared himself as the Son of God, a truth substantiated by several prophecies referencing the coming of the Son of God (Isa. 7:14, 9:6–7; Mic. 5:2). Despite the revelation, those hearing Jesus couldn't understand that He was the prophesied Son of God. Afterward, Jesus returned to the rural farmland with His family, continuing to honor and obey His parents. He remained steadfast in His commitment to follow the Mosaic laws and fulfill them (Matt. 5:17). Even though she couldn't grasp the full meaning of His words, Mary held all the extraordinary events in His life close to her heart. As time went on, more and more people recognized His divine wisdom and God's favor upon Him.

In certain prophecies, Jesus was referred to as the Son of God to highlight His divine nature, while in other Scriptures, He was named the Son of Man to signify His humanity (Dan. 7:13–14, 27; Ps. 80:17). He carried this dual title because he was fully God and fully human at the same time.

The ABC (Abstract to Brick Concrete)

Son of God—General Definition:[3]

- A superhuman or divine being (such as an angel); the expected king and deliverer of the Jews.

Son of God—Biblical Definition:

- A title signifying Jesus' deity and divine nature, portraying Him as the divine Son sent by God the Father to fulfill the mission of bringing salvation to humanity.

Son of Man—General Definition:[4]

- A human being; God's Messiah destined to preside over the final judgment of humankind.

Son of Man—Biblical Definition:

- A title illustrating the humanity of Jesus, highlighting that He possessed a fully human body and experienced the entirety of pain and suffering in all its forms.

---

3 "Son of God," Merriam-Webster.com, accessed October 23, 2023, https://www.merriam-webster.com.

4 "Son of Man," Merriam-Webster.com, accessed October 23, 2023, https://www.merriam-webster.com.

The FAST (Focused, Actionable Steps to Take)

1. Jesus, as the Son of God, triumphed over death through His resurrection, granting us eternal life and entry to the heavenly kingdom. We should value and treasure these precious gifts from Christ because, unlike earthly wealth, they are imperishable.

   Example: Peyton starts each day with prayers, expressing deep gratitude for the gift of eternal life and the promised entry into the heavenly kingdom. Every Thursday, she dedicates time to studying biblical passages about eternal life and the heavenly kingdom. During these sessions, Peyton examines herself, ensuring she remains steadfast, guarding against being led astray by the pursuit of earthly matters. This routine helps Peyton stay grounded in spiritual blessings, prioritizing eternal values over the transient allure of worldly treasures.

2. Jesus, as the Son of Man, bore the physical agony, emotional distress, and spiritual weight of humanity's sins during His crucifixion in His human form. Through His sacrifice, we found forgiveness, redemption, and reconciliation with God. His resurrection graciously granted us eternal life and entry into the heavenly kingdom. Communion is a ritual ceremony to remember the selfless sacrifice of Jesus. We, as Christians, share bread (symbolizing His body) and wine or grape juice (symbolizing His blood) to commemorate His crucifixion and death.

   Example: Shawn participates in the monthly communion at his church. As the communion elements pass through, he reflects deeply on the sacrifice Christ suffered for our salvation. Communion serves as a constant reminder of God's grace, motivating Shawn to practice forgiveness and love toward his fellow Christians.

APPENDIX

ABC Exercise Dictionary

Apostasy: A misleading belief system characterized by disregard for God, denial of Christ, and distortion of religious principles, often used to justify sinful behavior.

Bless: To bestow a temporal spiritual or earthly gift (how God blesses us); To worship and thank God for His mercies (how we bless God).

Calling: God's intended purpose of creation for the individual, accompanied by divine authority, guidance, and all the necessary attributes and provisions required to fulfill the assigned duty.

Child: An individual who, through faith, regardless of their social standing, past sins, or worldly labels, is embraced by God's love and grace, becoming a cherished member of His divine family.

Desperation: The driving force that compels one to risk everything in an attempt to seek God's attention, recognizing Him as the sole source of hope, a state of yearning for divine mercy.

Discernment: Having the capacity to distinguish between right and wrong, wise and foolish; to acquire an understanding of difficult or complex issues.

Drunkard: One who finds false security in deceptive and powerless entities like political alliances, false doctrines, and pagan idols.

Elect: One predestined for salvation and eternal life before the creation of the world; chosen by God, called through the work of the Holy Spirit, and justified through Christ.

Evangelism: The joyful proclamation of the message that salvation has come through Christ.

Faith:	The unwavering trust and belief in God's sacred covenants and divine characteristics, shielding Christians from temptations and deceit.
False Teachers:	Individuals whose teachings markedly deviate from canonical doctrines of Christianity.
Feast:	A moment of celebration where His people connect with God, unite as a community, and realign their lives and actions with His will.
Holy Ambition:	An unyielding desire to excel in fulfilling God's mission. This force of unity brings believers together through their shared goal of carrying out God's will.
Holy Zeal:	Unyielding determination to ensure that one's own actions do not obscure God's glory, but, instead, make it manifest to the entire world.
Hope	A robust, future-oriented confidence in Christ driving one toward their desired goals.
Hospitality:	A way of sharing the burdens of those serving God, recognizing that in doing so, we all work toward a common goal of serving God.
Idol:	Anything placed above one's allegiance to God.
Impiety:	Lacking true knowledge and understanding of God, often leading individuals to live in evil and wicked ways.
Judge:	To restore peace within a disrupted community, particularly for those who have suffered; to enact judgment on those responsible for the disruption; to rule as a means to exclude or even destroy those causing the disruption.
Justice:	A devoted pursuit for the divine will of God through wholehearted submission, transcending personal desires.
Law of Liberty:	A principle that liberates Christians from seeking righteousness through their own efforts and allows them to surpass the law's requirements through Christ's mercy.

APPENDIX: ABC Exercise Dictionary

Legacy:	An enduring impact and example set by devoted Christians, including their steadfast faith, commitment to Christian principles, and their practical application in daily life.
Loyal Love:	God's faithful love and kindness to His people.
Persecution:	An acknowledgment from the world of an individual's fulfillment of their divine mission.
Piety:	Possessing a knowledge and understanding of God, which can guide the individual to lead a righteous life.
Possession:	Divine blessings and responsibilities granted by God for our time on earth, to be managed with care and gratitude.
Reverence:	The fear of God, rooted in the belief in divine judgments, where the faithful are met with eternal blessings, and the evil receive lasting punishment.
Righteousness:	Displaying the qualities of Yahweh in one's words and actions; This involves living with compassion, extending grace, showing meekness, practicing love, upholding faithfulness, and standing for justice.
Revival:	A collective process of purging evil and wicked thoughts, feelings, and behaviors within a community, aiming to reestablish a connection with God.
Salvation:	Divine transformation of an individual's life, where through faith, they are reconciled with God and empowered to live a new, Christ-centered existence; shifting one's focus from worldly pursuits to a deep commitment to knowing, serving, and following Christ in their thoughts, actions, and relationships.
Sanctification:	The process guided by the Holy Spirit of detaching believers from the world's sway and transforming them into pure, spiritually mature, Christlike individuals.
Selfish Ambition:	An earthly, unspiritual, impure, and even demonic influence that incites evil actions and disrupts unity among believers.

Son of God:	A title signifying Jesus' deity and divine nature, portraying Him as the divine Son sent by God the Father to fulfill the mission of bringing salvation to humanity.
Son of Man:	A title illustrating the humanity of Jesus, highlighting that He possessed a fully human body and experienced the entirety of pain and suffering in all its forms.
Sovereignty:	The supreme and absolute authority of God over all creation, reflecting His unrivaled rulership and dominion.
Temple:	Each believer in whom God resides; relying on one's relationship with God rather than physical places.
Trial:	A challenging experience that tests one's faith, making it stronger as the individuals prepare themselves for eternal life in heaven.
Uncleanness:	Possessing a trait that God declared as unclean in the Old Testament; twisted by sinful individuals, religious teachers, and society into a reason to cruelly stigmatize, thus linked with pervasive bias and prejudice, resulting in heightened susceptibility to exclusion, discrimination, and mistreatment; the unclean were wrongly seen as "being" their uncleanness and having an impure identity; by the grace of God, the teachings of Christ redefined "uncleanness" as an opportunity for compassion, healing, and breaking down societal barriers.
Unity:	Oneness in harmony, driven by the shared purpose of serving Christ.
Vanity:	The pursuit of worldly success, wealth, and pleasure—which is empty and meaningless, since the only true fulfillment is found in a deeper relationship with God.
Wisdom:	Fear of God leading to the knowledge and skills needed to make the right choices for a successful, God-honoring life.

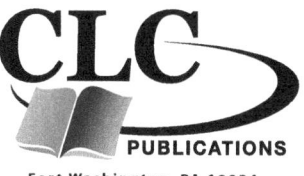

PUBLICATIONS
Fort Washington, PA 19034

This book is published by CLC Publications, an outreach of CLC Ministries International. The purpose of CLC is to make evangelical Christian literature available to all nations so that people may come to faith and maturity in the Lord Jesus Christ. We hope this book has been life changing and has enriched your walk with God through the work of the Holy Spirit. If you would like to know more about CLC, we invite you to visit our website:

www.clcusa.org

To know more about the remarkable story of the founding of CLC International we encourage you to read

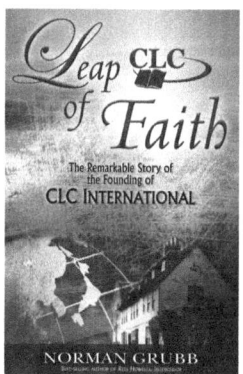

LEAP OF FAITH
Norman Grubb

Paperback
Size 5¼ x 8, Pages 248
ISBN: 978-0-87508-650-7
ISBN (*e-book*): 978-1-61958-055-8

Also from CLC Publications

Becoming a Worthy Reader
How to Read and Study the Bible

Kevin D. Zuber

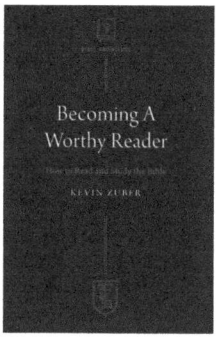

"I delight in your decrees; I will not neglect your word." (Ps. 119:16)

How can Christians grow in biblical literacy, deepening their understanding and application of Scripture?

Kevin D. Zuber teaches hermeneutics, the process of correctly reading and interpreting Scripture, in an accessible way. Correcting common errors, Zuber provides a guide that helps Christians navigate the genres and contexts of the Bible. Zuber not only enriches Christians' understanding of Wisdom, Apocalyptic, and Prophetic literature, but also empowers Christians to become worthy scholars of God's Word with the help of the Spirit.

Learn to move beyond trite and questionable interpretations of Scripture and mature into a worthy scholar of the Bible!

Part of the Institute for the Christian Life Series

Paperback
Size 6 x 9, Pages 224
ISBN 978-1-61958-382-5
ISBN (*e-book*) 978-1-61958-383-2

Blurry
Bringing Clarity to the Bible

Ryan Lokkesmoe

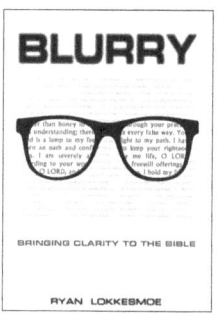

Do you want a better understanding of the Bible but don't know where to start? Do you want a clear perspective of how the whole Bible fits together? *Blurry: Bringing Clarity to the Bible* is for YOU!

Ryan Lokkesmoe offers a brief, yet innovative, introduction to the Bible in plain language. Highlighting four books, Genesis, Luke, Ephesians, and James, Blurry brings the Bible into focus with easy-to-use reading strategies, charts, and group discussion questions. No insider language. No cryptic diagrams. No theological speeches. Blurry is a straightforward set of first steps that will propel you into a lifetime of reading and enjoying the Bible.

> "Whether you're a long-time Christian or just starting out on your journey, Ryan Lokkesmoe has put together a helpful and straightforward introduction to the Bible. I encourage you to read it for yourself and then pass it on to a friend."
> —Larry Osborne, Author and Pastor
> North Coast Church, Vista, CA

Paperback
Size 5.25 x 8, Pages 154
ISBN 978-1-61958-164-7
ISBN (*e-book*) 978-1-61958-165-4